DIETARY FIBRE
MECHANISMS OF ACTION
IN HUMAN PHYSIOLOGY AND METABOLISM

British Library Cataloguing in Publication Data
A catalogue record for this book is available from the British Library.

ISBN 2-7420-0096-8

Éditions John Libbey Eurotext
127, avenue de la République, 92120 Montrouge, France
Tél. : (1) 46.73.06.60

John Libbey and Company Ltd
13, Smiths Yard, Summerley Street,
London SW18 4HR, England
Tel. : (1) 947.27.77

John Libbey CIC
Via L. Spallanzani, 11
00161, Rome, Italy
Tel. : (06) 862.289

© 1995, John Libbey Eurotext, Paris

Il est interdit de reproduire intégralement ou partiellement le présent ouvrage — loi du 11 mars 1957 — sans autorisation de l'éditeur ou du Centre Français du Copyright, 6 *bis*, rue Gabriel-Laumain, 75010 Paris, France.

DIETARY FIBRE
MECHANISMS OF ACTION IN HUMAN PHYSIOLOGY AND METABOLISM

Proceedings of an international conference organised by the EU COST 92 programme Nantes (France), June 20-22, 1994

Edited by

C. CHERBUT
J.L. BARRY
D. LAIRON
M. DURAND

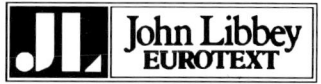

Illustration de couverture :
Pains quotidiens. Herman BRAUN - VEGA, 1993.
Photo : Patrice MAURIN BERTHIER.

Contents

List of contributors VII

Foreword VIII

Preface
   C. Cherbut, J.L. Barry, D. Lairon, M. Durand IX

Dietary fibre : do we still have an hypothesis to test ?
   J.H. Cummings 1

Physico-chemical properties of dietary fibre in the foregut
   M. Eastwood 17

Fermentation of polysaccharides by human colonic anaerobes
   A.A. Salyers 29

The production of short-chain fatty acids in the human colon
   P.B. Mortensen, I. Nordgaard 37

Dietary fibre, fermentation and the colon
   C.A. Edwards 51

Effects of short-chain fatty acids on gastro-intestinal epithelial cells
   T. Sakata 61

Dietary fibre and lipid metabolism in humans
   T.M.S. Wolever 69

Fibre effect on nutrient metabolism in splanchnic and peripheral tissues.
   B. Darcy-Vrillon, P.H. Duée 83

List of contributors

Cummings J.H., Dunn Clinical Nutrition Centre, Hills Road, Cambridge CB2 2DH, UK.

Darcy-Vrillon B., Unité d'Écologie et de Physiologie du Système Digestif, Institut National de la Recherche Agronomique, 78352 Jouy-en-Josas Cedex, France.

Duée P., Unité d'Écologie et de Physiologie du Système Digestif, Institut National de la Recherche Agronomique, 78352 Jouy-en-Josas Cedex, France.

Eastwood M., Gastrointestinal Unit, Western General Hospital, Edinburgh EH4 2XU, UK.

Edwards C.A., Department of Human Nutrition, Glasgow University, Yorkhill Hospitals, Glasgow G3 8SJ, UK.

Mortensen P.B., University of Copenhagen, Department of Medicine A-2151, Division of Gastroenterology and Hepatology, Rigshospitalet, 9 Blegdamsvej, DK-2100 Copenhagen, Denmark.

Nordgaard I., University of Copenhagen, Department of Medicine A-2151, Division of Gastroenterology and Hepatology, Rigshospitalet, 9 Blegdamsvej, DK-2100 Copenhagen, Denmark.

Sakata T., Department of Basic Sciences, Ishinomaki Senshu University, Minamisakai Shinmito 1, Ishinomaki 986, Miyagi, Japan.

Salyers A.A, Department of Microbiology, University of Illinois, Urbana, IL 61801, USA.

Wolever T.M.S., Department of Nutritional Sciences, 150 College Street, University of Toronto, Toronto, Ontario, Canada M55 1A8.

Foreword

It is now almost 25 years since Burkitt noted that « the close relationship between bowel cancer and other non-infective diseases ...and... their close association with the refined diet characteristic of economic development suggests that the removal of dietary fibre may be the causative factor ». This hypothesis was subsequently expanded by Trowel, Walker and others to encompass many of the major diseases of Western culture including coronary heart disease, obesity, diabetes, gall stones and other bowel disorders. None of these early pioneers actually measured fibre in the diet or intakes in any population, and whilst proposing an exciting concept, they have left us with a confusion of definitions and methodologies.

Despite this, the dietary fibre hypothesis has been one of the most compelling in nutrition and public health in the latter half of the twentieth century. It has provided the stimulus to a great deal of research both epidemiological, physiological, analytical and technical. It has been the catalyst for rapid progress in our understanding of the cause of a number of common diseases, especially those of the large bowel, and given governments and the food industry valuable targets for healthy eating.

Biological science has progressed in many ways in recent years, and this is reflected in current fibre research as presented in this conference report. Fibre, through its fermentation, is now known to effect the growth and differentiation of epithelial cells in the gut, hepatic metabolism of carbohydrate and lipid, and genotoxic events within the large bowel. The physical properties of fibre have proved difficult to study, but are essential to its role in moderating glucose and insulin responses in the blood. The breakdown of fibre by the colonic bacteria has given new insights into their importance for health.

Fibre has thus facilitated a broadening of our understanding of gut physiology and metabolism and has identified the colon as a major digestive organ. Fibre research has let to a re-appraisal of the digestive physiology of other carbohydrates, particularly starches and oligosaccharides which may be equally important in protecting against Western diseases.

The Management Committee of COST 92, which was set up in 1990, now includes delegates from fifteen European countries which has as its aim to study and co-ordinate activities related to the « Metabolic and Physiological Aspects of Dietary Fibre ». This it has done by sponsoring a series of workshops and the first international conference of dietary fibre, promoted by the Human Nutrition Research Centre of Nantes. The focus of this meeting has been « mechanisms of action » and it is clear from these proceedings that fibre research is a very productive area in Europe, of great interest to agriculture, the food industry, nutrition and medicine.

John H. Cummings
Dunn Clinical Nutrition Centre
Cambridge

March 1995

Preface

The international conference held on 20-22 June 1994 in Nantes, France, within the framework of the European Union COST 92 programme (Metabolic and physiological aspects of dietary fibre in foods) was the third in a series which began on 1990 in Norwich (UK), where « Biochemical and biological aspects of dietary fibre » were discussed and continued on 1992 with « Topics in dietary fibre » in Roma (Italy).

During the past two decades, an extensive description of many physiological and metabolic effects of dietary fibre has been achieved. However, the mechanisms of the fibre action are still uncompletely clarified. The Nantes' conference aimed at improving the understanding of these mechanisms, which required to bring together researchers from disciplines as different as Food Science, Nutrition, Gastroenterology, Endocrinology, Cell Biology, Microbiology, etc. This book is the result of their productive discussion. It is built from the main papers presented by leading scientists and should provide an up-to-date synthesis of the current knowledge about the action of dietary fibre in man. We warmly thank all the contributors.

The Nantes' conference was held under the auspice of the European Union and was also supported by the French Ministry of High Education and Research (MESR), the National Institute for Agricultural Research (INRA), the National Institute for Health and Medical Research (INSERM) and the « Pays-de-Loire » district : we are pleased to thank all of them. We are also grateful to the sponsors who brought us financial help.

We extend our thanks to A. Scherer, M. Chapeau and G. Nicol, from the Nantes INRA Centre, for their patient and effective help.

Above all, we would like to thank all those who attended the conference and made it successful.

C. Cherbut, J.L. Barry, D. Lairon and M. Durand

1

Dietary fibre : do we still have an hypothesis to test ?

J.H. CUMMINGS

*Dunn Clinical Nutrition Centre, Hills Road,
Cambridge, CB2 2DH, UK*

Evolution of the fibre concept

The dietary fibre concept became known in the early 1970's as a result of the convergence of evidence from epidemiology, physiology and analytical studies [1-5]. This concept related the nature of diet to the prevalence of coronary heart disease, obesity, diabetes, gallstones and various conditions of the large bowel.

Epidemiology

Although much had already been written about fibre, the first epidemiological observations of importance were probably those of Higginson and Oettlé in 1960 who noted that constipation and bowel cancer were rare in Africa whilst being common in the West, and that in Africa « a large amount of roughage is consumed... » and « stools are bulkier and more frequent... » [6, 7]. In 1971, Burkitt [8] suggested a specific hypothesis relating lack of dietary fibre to the cause of bowel cancer and a mechanism whereby fibre, through its capacity to « regulate the speed of transit, bulk and consistency of stool.... » and effect microbial metabolism was able to prevent bowel cancer.

About this time, Trowell, influenced by his experience in Uganda, which he had summarised in his book *Non-infective diseases in Africa* [9], and by reading Cleave's *... The Saccharine Disease* [10], suggested that a number of other chronic Western diseases such as obesity, diabetes, coronary heart disease, gallstones, etc. might also be due to consumption of fibre-depleted foods. Concurrently, Painter, working in Oxford, proposed that diverticular disease was due to colonic stasis induced by lack of fibre [11, 12]. Burkitt and Walker then added varicose veins and haemorrhoids to the list of fibre-deficiency disorders [13].

Physiology

Parallel with these epidemiological observations was the development of knowledge of the physiological properties of fibre in the gut. The polysaccharides of the plant cell wall were thought not to be digested in the upper intestine of man, but to be fermented in the large bowel by bacteria and thus increase stool output, shorten transit time, alter bile acid metabolism and produce volatile fatty acids [2]. A number of animal studies had shown cholesterol lowering and atheroma preventing effects of fibre [2] and in man the beneficial effect of oats [14] and pectin [15] was already known.

Methods

Advances were also occurring at this time in methods for determination of dietary fibre in the laboratory [16-18], most notable of which were those of Southgate [16], and in animal nutrition, of Van Soest [19].

Definition

The convergence of these three lines of evidence gave birth and credence to the dietary fibre concept and stimulated Burkitt and Trowell to prepare to write a book [1]. Burkitt wrote to Trowell asking him to define « dietary fibre ». Trowell thought this would be simple but could not find fibre defined in any textbooks of medicine or nutrition [20]. Some food tables listed values for the crude fibre content of foods. Crude fibre, a gravimetric method used to analyse animal feeds, had been in use for over 150 years. However, Van Soest and colleagues had already shown that this method failed to recover the majority of the plant cell wall material [19].

In the United Kingdom, the Medical Research Council's « Composition of Foods » [21] contained data on « unavailable carbohydrate », a term used by McCance and Lawrence in 1929 [22] and earlier by Atwater. In trying to prepare accurate food tables for diabetic diets, McCance and Lawrence tried to distinguish between « available carbohydrate consists of starch and soluble sugars... and the ... unavailable, mainly... hemicellulose and fibre (cellulose) ».

Trowell, however, wanted a generic term for the undigested plant cell wall that he thought was important to health and so he decided to redefine fibre [20]. The earliest formal description of dietary fibre was therefore by Trowell who defined it as « the proportion of food which is derived from the cellular walls of plants which is digested very poorly in human beings » [23]. This was largely an attempt to distinguish it from crude fibre. It was a physiological-botanical definition which did not identify the precise nature of dietary fibre nor define exactly the limiting characteristics of substances that should be included or excluded in the description, apart from the reference to plant cell wall material. Moreover, there was no method specified.

Subsequently Trowell discovered that Hipsley [24] had used the term « dietary fibre » in an article on pregnancy toxaemia, stating it was cellulose, hemicellulose and lignin. However, his paper contained data on crude fibre.

After visiting the USA in 1974, Trowell [25] enlarged his definition of dietary fibre to include structural polysaccharides, lignins, unavailable lipids, nitrogen, trace elements and cell wall « enzymes and mineral salts ». This was really an acknowledgement that the concept of fibre and disease could not be ascribed to any particular cell wall component at that time.

In 1976, in conjunction with Southgate, Wolever, Leeds, Gassull and Jenkins, fibre was redefined as « the plant polysaccharides and lignin which are resistant to hydrolysis by the digestive enzymes of man » [26]. This definition was specifically chosen so that polysaccharides structurally related to plant cell wall polysaccharides would be included in the definition. These isolated polysaccharides were being used experimentally to investigate the physiological effects of dietary fibre. More pragmatically, the isolated polysaccharides were also analytically indistinguishable from the corresponding plant cell wall components.

Since 1976, both Trowell and many others have defined and redefined dietary fibre. However, what has emerged from analytical, physiological and epidemiological studies is that the health benefits of fibre are conferred primarily by the polysaccharides of the plant cell wall, namely cellulose, hemicellulose and pectin as a result of their chemical and physical properties which in turn lead to specific physiological changes [27-31]. No other plant cell wall component has been shown to be important in man in the context of preventing Western diseases, although other dietary constituents such as resistant starch, oligosaccharides and lignin may contribute to or modify these effects. The cell wall polysaccharides are a chemically distinct group of carbohydrates, which do not contain the alphaglucosidic bonds present in starch and they have been called non-starch polysaccharides (NSP) [32, 33]. The amount of NSP in the diet is quantitatively related to bowel function [34]. This latter property has formed the basis for dietary recommendations for fibre intakes in both the UK and WHO recently [35, 36].

So where does the dietary fibre hypothesis stand today ? The early papers of Burkitt and colleagues have stimulated a great deal of research. Prior to 1970, there are very few papers on dietary fibre, less than five per year. By 1980, around 300 papers were being published annually on this topic, and in 1990, the number was around 500.

Fibre research in Europe

Recently, the Management Committee of COST 92 completed a survey of dietary fibre research activities in Europe in order to identify the strengths and weaknesses overall of European work in this field. Twenty seven research areas were identified, in which over 250 individual projects were being carried out in the 14 countries from which information was compiled. The most popular areas for research, in order, are cholesterol, lipid and coronary heart disease ; fermentation and short chain fatty acids ; mineral absorption, phytate and antinutrients ; and analysis and characterisation of dietary fibre. This emphasis in activities is reflected in publications over this period with about 14 % of the total on the topic of measurement and analysis, 12 % on lipids and heart disease, and 10 % on fermentation. What was evident from the survey, however, was the lack of research effort in dietary fibre epidemiology and intakes, which is surprising since such information is essential to establishing the potential role for health of dietary fibre. Some clinical topics were also poorly covered, for example the effects of fibre on appetite, pancreatic function, hepatic metabolism, cellular metabolism and proliferation in the large bowel, and gallstone formation. In other areas, at least ten groups are active [37].

Some of the diseases on the original list of fibre-deficiency disorders have fallen by the wayside. These include gallstones, varicose veins, hiatus hernia, irritable bowel, appendicitis and haemorrhoids, largely because other better theories have been advocated, or little research has been targeted at these fields. For appetite and obesity, lipids and coronary heart disease, carbohydrates and diabetes, and large bowel disorders, much work has been done and some judgement can be made of the real importance of fibre.

Appetite, satiety and obesity

Many studies have been reported of the effect of various sources of NSP on both short term appetite and satiety and long term weight changes. NSP-rich foods are generally less energy dense, more bulky and it is not unreasonable to suppose they may affect appetite. *Table I* summarises the results from 17 reports of 20 short term studies on appetite and show that the majority, 15 out of 20, observed a reduction in hunger. It is of course easy to criticise these studies because of the difficulty in blinding either subjects or investigators to the food being consumed. Moreover, to allow valid changes in food intake under experimental conditions to occur, when appetite is subject to so many physiological, psychological and social controls, is difficult. Nevertheless, there is a feeling amongst researchers in this field that NSP containing foods or supplements may be satiating.

Turning short term satiety into long term weight control is another matter, and as *Table II* shows, the results of such studies are less clear. A major problem in long term studies is of course compliance, particularly in the obese. Moreover, physiological adaptation may occur to changes in energy intake.

There are no good epidemiological studies of obesity and NSP intake, but some potential mechanisms exist. NSP, by virtue of its physical properties, may delay

Table I. Short term studies of fibre and appetite (n = 17). (From [38, 39].)

Source	n	Amount	Hunger	
			Reduced	No change
Methylcellulose	3	1 to 3	2	1
Guar	5	2 to 8	3	2
Guar/Bran	1	12	1	0
Bran	3	6	2	1
Alginate	1	2+	1	0
Fruit	2	14 to 16	2	0
Mixed sources	5	7 to 39	4	1
		Total	15	5

gastric emptying, produce increased bulk in the upper gut and regulate carbohydrate and lipid absorption. However, in the large intestine, the fermentation of NSP produces short chain fatty acids (SCFA) which in turn provide energy. Evidence from animal studies do not provide a role for SCFA in controlling appetite [40].

Overall therefore NSP containing foods or supplements show a reduction in appetite in short term studies but no consistent change in energy balance long term. Some possible mechanisms have been described affecting the upper gut but NSP is a source of energy through fermentation. Many other factors contribute to the control of appetite and weight. NSP is probably not the principal one.

Lipids and coronary heart disease

It is now well established that certain forms of non-starch polysaccharide can lower blood cholesterol in man. This was shown as far back as 1961 [15] and the many subsequent studies have been reviewed extensively [41, 42]. In summary, they show that soluble forms of NSP, such as pectin and guar gum and the soluble β-glucans in oats, lower blood cholesterol in healthy and hyperlipidaemic subjects. Insoluble NSP, such as that present in wheat bran or pure cellulose, do not usually have this effect. The possible mechanisms whereby NSP may lower blood cholesterol are several and not yet conclusively decided. They include an effect of the water-soluble gel-forming materials in inhibiting cholesterol absorption in the small intestine, or affecting bile acid absorption and metabolism. Also soluble NSP is readily fermented in the large intestine producing short chain fatty acids, including propionic acid. There are some *in vitro* and animal and human studies to show that propionic acid may be hypocholesterolaemic [43-47]. Finally, soluble NSP has notable effects on blood glucose and insulin metabolism *(see below)* and, through this, may also indirectly affect lipoprotein metabolism and the clotting system [48].

Although an association between coronary heart disease and dietary fibre was suggested in the 1950's [49, 50], few recent epidemiological attempts have been made to correlate « fibre » intake with heart disease risk. Temporal correlation studies have not provided convincing evidence for a protective effect of fibre and these studies can be criticised for the nature of the fibre intake data that is used. Mostly only very imprecise intake measurements have been made and there are really no good cross-sectional studies using accurate measurements of NSP intake.

Table II. Long term studies of fibre and obesity (n = 20). (From [37, 38].)

Source	n	Amount g/day	Duration (weeks)	Weight loss	
				Yes	No
Guar/glucomannan	4	15 to 20	1 to 18	4	0
Cellulose	1	30	—	0	1
Methylcellulose	3	4 to 16	to 21	1	3
Bran/mixed	5	6 to 40	1 to 56	2	2
Mixed	7	5 to 15	to 60	5	2
			Total	12	8

A number of prospective studies have been done of diet and heart disease and these show a much more consistently protective effect of fibre. These include the studies of Morris *et al.* [51] in London, Yano *et al.* [52] in Honolulu, the Zutphen study [53] and the Boston-Irish study [54]. In all these, some measure of total « fibre » intake has been made and the coronary heart disease cases have had uniformly lower intakes. However, the results are confounded by the close inter-association between dietary patterns which reflect high fat, low carbohydrate and vice-versa. In Morris *et al.*'s study [51], the protective relationship was with cereals not vegetables and fruit, whilst the protective effect of crude fibre in the Boston-Irish study [54] was not significant when adjusted for other risk factors. Similarly in the Zutphen study [53], the significant inverse relationship between coronary heart disease mortality and fibre disappeared with multivariate analysis. This study did show a protective effect for polysaccharide consumption and, in both the Honolulu heart study [52] and a study in Puerto Rico [55], starch intakes were apparently protective. There is a clear need for more work to be done using good methods of dietary intake assessment and precise measurements of all the carbohydrates in the diet.

Perhaps the most important thing about coronary heart disease is that it is a condition in which there are a number of cellular and pathological events which lead

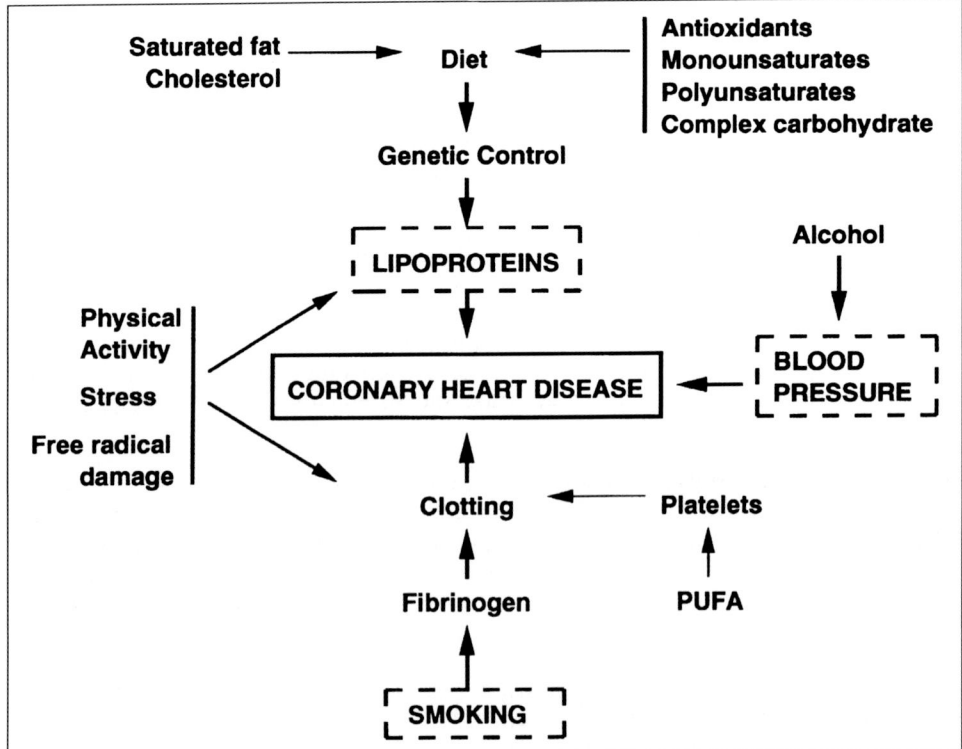

Figure 1. Major risk factors and other contributory causes to coronary heart disease. Modified from [56].

ultimately to coronary occlusion and often to death. The major risk factors are a raised blood pressure, raised serum cholesterol and smoking. A number of other processes also relate to risk in this condition and these are summarised in *Figure 1*. From *Figure 1*, it can readily be seen that diet itself is only one of a number of causes contributing to risk of coronary heart disease and furthermore that fibre is only one of the many dietary components which effect risk.

Overall therefore with regard to fibre and coronary heart disease, we have a multifactorial problem for which there is some evidence for a contribution from fibre. Soluble forms of NSP usually lower blood cholesterol and there may be effects on the clotting system as well. Insoluble forms of NSP are not however generally regarded as hypocholesterolaemic. Prospective epidemiological studies show a protective effect for diets characterised by high fibre intakes and a number of physiological mechanisms exist which relate these events. « Fibre » or more probably NSP has a significant contributory, but not major, role in the aetiology of coronary heart disease.

Glucose, insulin and diabetes

To Trowell must go the credit for first identifying a link between fibre and diabetes [57, 58], and to Jenkins and colleagues for publishing the first experimental evidence in man that fibre moderated blood glucose and insulin responses [59]. Since then, recommendations for the diabetic diet have changed from a low carbohydrate high fat high protein diet to one moderately low in fat and high in starch and NSP [60, 61].

The subject has been extensively researched and evidence is summarised in recent reviews [62, 63]. Guar gum has probably been most studied and, as Wolever and Jenkins point out (63), an average reduction of 44 % in blood glucose was seen in 15 studies of 24 groups of people with guar. In a similar meta-analysis, pectin reduced blood glucose by 29 % and psyllium 29 % also. Jenkins pointed out at an early stage that it was primarily soluble sources of NSP which formed gels, which were most effective in this context [64].

However, events have overtaken the soluble dietary fibre story in diabetes. Long term studies of soluble fibre use highlighted a number of problems of acceptability, side effects, dose, etc. Equally good effects in diabetes could be achieved by diets high in starchy foods [65] and the nature of these starchy foods influenced blood glucose [66, 67]. The concept of the glycaemic index was born [68] and a whole new area of nutritional science has developed, which has concerned itself with glycaemic responses to carbohydrate and other foods. The major factors now known to control blood glucose response to normal foods in healthy people are summarised in *Table III*. The nature of the starch is the key and the subject of much current intensive research [69, 70].

Despite this interest in starch, there may still be a unique role for NSP in the control of carbohydrate metabolism. The early studies of viscosity and glucose responses pointed to the physical properties of NSP as being important. The classic study of Haber *et al.* [71] with apples shows clearly that where carbohydrate, in this case sugar, is entrapped intracellularly in plant foods, its release in the gut

Table III. Major factors affecting blood glucose and insulin responses.

Starch	Physical form
	Granule structure
	Gelatinisation state
	Amylose/amylopectin ratio
NSP	Physical structure
	Viscosity
Fat/protein	
Phytate/lectins/transit rate, etc.	
Amount of carbohydrate	

is slowed and blood glucose and insulin responses lowered. The unique property of NSP therefore is that it forms the plant cell wall and thus a physical structure to foods. Numerous studies have now shown that the physical structure of starchy foods determines glycaemic index.

NSP may therefore have a role to play in the regulation of carbohydrate metabolism through the physical structure it imparts to foods. The use of viscous soluble NSP isolates in this context will probably be seen as a stepping stone to understanding fibre but not the ultimate goal. In trying to understand the dietary control of blood glucose and insulin, however, it is essential to start with a study of all carbohydrate, of which NSP is a part.

Table IV. Effect of NSP in the large intestine.

	Effect	Disease
Unfermented (*e.g.* wheat bran)	Bulk	Constipation
Fermented		
• Short chain fatty acids		
Acetate	Energy source	—
Proprionate	Uptake in liver	Coronary heart disease
	Cholesterol metabolism	
Butyrate	Epithelial metabolism	Cancer, colitis
• H_2, CO_2, CH_4	Hydrogen metabolism	Pneumatosis cystoides intestinalis
• Biomass	Bulk	Laxation
	Bacterial protein synthesis	Carcinogen metabolism

Table V. Molar ratios of short chain fatty acids from fermentation of NSP.

Source	Acetate	Propionate	Butyrate	References
Pectin	80	11	9	[83-89]
Arabinogalactan	57	31	12	[83, 84, 88, 89]
Psyllium	73	15	12	[85, 90]
Guar	59	28	13	[85, 86, 91]
Oat bran	61	16	21	[84, 91]
Wheat bran	62	17	21	[84, 86, 91]
Soya	69	21	10	[85, 87]

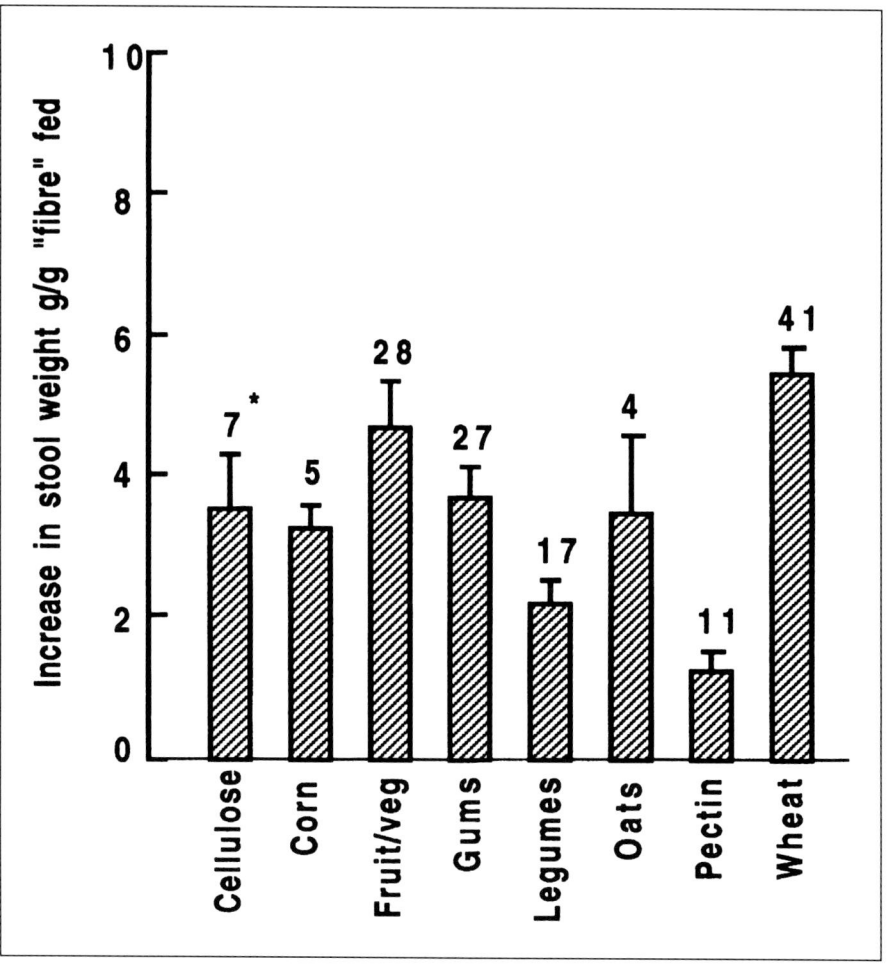

Figure 2. Average increase in stool wet weight per gram « dietary fibre » fed from various sources. Results are from 140 published studies (*Number studies used to calculate average and SEM). From [74].

Fermentation and the large intestine

It is now well established that NSP reaches the large intestine and is fermented with the production of SCFA, H_2, CO_2 and biomass [72]. This fermentative process dominates human large bowel function and provides a means whereby energy can be salvaged from carbohydrate not digested in the small bowel, through absorption of SCFA. The physiological consequences of fermentation are diverse and are summarised in *Table IV*. Several have important implications for human diseases.

The best known effect is that on bowel habit. Many hundreds of papers have been published on this subject and the key ones are summarised in [73]. *Figure 2* is a compilation of faecal weight data from around 120 papers published between 1932 and 1992 detailing 150 separate studies. It shows the average increase in stool output expressed as grams of stool (wet weight) per gram of « fibre » fed. Studies were included only if they contained quantitative data on changes in stool weight and had at least one control and one test period.

Wheat as a source comes out as the most effective at 5.4 (0.7 SEM) g stool/g fibre fed as averaged from 41 studies. Raw bran at 7.2 g/g is more effective than cooked bran, 4.9 ($p < 0,05$), but has the disadvantage of containing 3 % phytate — a known inhibitor of the absorption of divalent cations (calcium, magnesium, zinc and iron). Fruit and vegetables are remarkably effective, 4.7 (0.7) g/g, and with wheat are well ahead of the rest. Whilst many people believe fruit and vegetables to contain mainly soluble NSP, in fact this is not the case. They contain significant amounts of insoluble NSP and moreover most of these laxative studies were done using whole foods containing intact plant cell walls, which probably contributes to their effect. After fruit and vegetables come gums and mucilages at 3.7 (0.5) g/g. This includes most of the bulk laxatives *(see later)*. The league table then progresses through cellulose 3.5 (0.8), oats 3.4 (1.1), corn 3.3 (0.3), legumes (mainly soya) 2.2 (0.3) and lastly pectin 1.2 (0.3).

How reliable are these rankings ? Within each group, there is great variability, although despite this, the overall differences are statistically significant (by ANOVAR F 4.78 $p < 0.001$). The variability is due in part to the inherent difference in individual responses and to varying experimental designs, some of which are uncontrolled diets. A further problem is lack of consistency in methodology for measurement of dietary fibre. Around 20 different methods were used in these studies, some of which give only a rough approximation of the true NSP content of the food or source. These laxative properties of NSP are used in the prevention and treatment of constipation [74].

The principal products of fermentation are the SCFA, acetate, propionate and butyrate. Their physiological and clinical importance are reviewed in two recent books [75, 76]. Each SCFA has different properties. Acetate is absorbed and reaches the peripheral circulation where it is taken up by muscle and metabolised as an energy source. Propionate is partly cleared by the colonic epithelium and then very largely by the liver. It may be important in the control of cholesterol metabolism *(see above)*. Butyrate has attracted a great deal of attention because of its role as an energy source for the epithelium [77, 78] and its effects on cell growth and differentiation [79-81]. These are reviewed elsewhere in this Symposium and in [82].

NSP are an important source of SCFA. Since however each fatty acid has its own properties, the relative amounts produced from a source of NSP will in turn determine its physiological role. *In vitro* studies of NSP fermentation have shown that the molar proportions of fatty acids produced may vary from one source of NSP to another. *Table V* summarises a number of published studies. In all cases, acetate is the major anion comprising 67 % overall of total SCFA. Pectin is a particularly good source of acetate (81 % in 7 studies), whilst arabinogalactan (54 % n = 3) and guar (59 % n = 3) are the poorest sources. By contrast, guar and arabinogalactan are good sources of propionate (27 % and 34 % respectively). Butyrate production varies over a wide range. Perhaps the most important development about butyrate relates to its potential to protect against large bowel cancer [82].

Many other aspects of fermentation are covered elsewhere in this Symposium. However, it is important to remember that NSP is not the only substrate. A number of other carbohydrates reach the large intestine including resistant starches, oligosaccharides, some sugars and sugar alcohols. The role of NSP in fermentation is therefore not unique but nevertheless it is a major contributor to bowel function.

Conclusion

The dietary fibre hypothesis was in many ways revolutionary and has stimulated a great deal of research in the ensuing 20 years. During this time, knowledge has increased and a number of more definitive hypotheses have emerged. There is now a good experimental basis to link fibre with the control of bowel habit and the prevention of constipation. There is also evidence from epidemiological, animal and human studies to support the view that fibre will contribute to the prevention of bowel cancer, moderate carbohydrate absorption and so be beneficial in the dietary management of diabetes and similarly with lipid absorption and coronary heart disease. Such properties are of direct importance to public health, particularly in the prevention of bowel diseases.

However, it is clear that a number of other dietary components contribute to the aetiology of these diseases and that fibre may not be the major factor in any of them. Moreover fibre has not been shown to have any unique properties in the gut other than its physical effects, and cannot on its own explain the aetiology of any Western disease, even constipation. Twenty years of research have therefore shown that the original dietary fibre hypothesis is incomplete, but the concept has provided a valuable stimulus to research into the understanding of many Western diseases.

References

1. Burkitt DP, Trowell HS. *Refined carbohydrate foods and disease : some implications of dietary fibre.* London, New York : Academic Press, 1975.
2. Cummings JH. Dietary fibre : progress report. *Gut* 1973 ; 14 : 69-81.
3. Symposium on « Fibre in Human Nutrition ». *Proc Nutr Soc* 1973 ; 32 : 123-67.
4. Reilly RW, Kirsner JB. Fiber deficiency and colonic disorders. New York : Plenum, 1975.
5. Painter NS. *Diverticular disease of the colon. A deficiency disease of Western civilization.* London : William Heinemann Medical Books, 1975.
6. Higginson J, Oettle AG. Cancer incidence in the Bantu and « Cape Colored » races of

South Africa : report of a cancer survey in the Transvaal (1953-55). *J Natl Cancer Inst* 1960 ; 24 : 589-671.
7. Oettle AG. Cancer in Africa, especially in regions South of the Sahara. *J Natl Cancer Inst* 1964 ; 33 : 383-439.
8. Burkitt DP. Epidemiology of cancer of the colon and rectum. *Cancer* 1971 ; 28 : 3-13.
9. Trowell HC. *Non-infective diseases in Africa*. London : Edward Arnold, 1960.
10. Cleave TL. *The saccharine disease*. Bristol : John Wright, 1974.
11. Painter NS. Diverticular disease of the colon : a disease of this century. *Lancet* 1969 ; 2 : 586-8.
12. Painter NS, Burkitt DP. Diverticular disease of the colon : a deficiency disease of Western civilisation. *Br Med J* 1971 ; 2 : 450-4.
13. Burkitt DP, Walker ARP, Painter NS. Effect of dietary fibre on stools and transit times, and its role in the causation of disease. *Lancet* 1972 ; ii : 1408-12.
14. Groot AP de, Luyken R, Pikaar NA. Cholesterol-lowering effect of rolled oats. (Letter). *Lancet* 1963 ; 2 : 303-4.
15. Keys A, Grande F, Anderson JT. Fiber and pectin in the diet and serum cholesterol concentration in man. *Proc Soc Exp Biol (NY)* 1961 ; 106 : 555-8.
16. Southgate DAT. Determination of carbohydrates in foods. II. Unavailable carbohydrates. *J Sci Food Agric* 1969 ; 20 : 331-5.
17. Thomas M. *Die Nahr und Ballastoffe der Getreidemehle in ihrer Bedeutung fur die Brotnahrung*. Stuttgart : Wissenschaftliche Verlagsgesellschaft, 1964.
18. Hellendoorn EW, Noordhoff MG, Slagman J. Enzymatic determination of the indigestible residue (dietary fibre) content of human food. *J Sci Food Agric* 1975 ; 26 : 1461-8.
19. Van Soest PJ, McQueen RW. The chemistry and estimation of fibre. *Proc Nutr Soc* 1973 ; 32 : 123-30.
20. Trowell H. Dietary fibre : a paradigm. In : Trowell H, Burkitt D, Heaton KW, eds. *Dietary fibre, fibre-depleted foods and disease*. London : Academic Press, 1985 : 1-20.
21. McCance RA, Widdowson EM. *The Chemical composition of foods*. London : HMSO (special report series of the Medical Research Council, No. 235), 1940.
22. McCance RA, Lawrence RD. *The carbohydrate content of foods*. London : HMSO (special report series of the Medical Research Council, No. 135), 1929.
23. Trowell H. Dietary fibre and coronary heart disease. *Eur J Clin Biol Res* 1972 ; 17 : 345-9.
24. Hipsley EH. Dietary « fibre » and pregnancy toxaemia. *Br Med J* 1953 ; ii : 420-2.
25. Trowell H. Definitions of fibre. (Letter). *Lancet* 1974 ; i : 503.
26. Trowell H, Southgate DAT, Wolever TMS, Leeds AR, Gassull MA, Jenkins DJA. Dietary fibre redefined. (Letter). *Lancet* 1976 ; i : 967.
27. Kritchevsky D, Bonfield C, Anderson JW. *Dietary fiber. Chemistry, physiology and health effects*. New York : Plenum Press, 1990.
28. Southgate DAT, Waldron K, Johnson IT, Fenwick GR. *Dietary fibre : chemical and biological aspects*. Royal Society of Chemistry, 1990.
29. Schweizer TF, Edwards CA. *Dietary fibre. A component of food ; nutritional function in health and disease*. London : Springer Verlag, 1992.
30. Pilch SM. *Physiological effects and health consequences of dietary fiber*. Maryland, USA : Life Sciences Research Office, 1987.
31. British Nutrition Foundation. *Complex carbohydrates in foods*. Report of the British Nutrition Foundation's Task Force. Chapman & Hall, 1990.
32. Cummings JH. Some aspects of dietary fibre metabolism in the human gut. In : Birch GA, ed. *Food and Health. Science and technology*. London : Applied Science Publishers Ltd., 1980 : 441-58.
33. Englyst HN, Trowell H, Southgate DAT, Cummings JH. Dietary fiber and resistant starch. *Am J Clin Nutr* 1987 ; 46 : 873-4.
34. Cummings JH, Bingham SA, Heaton KW, Eastwood MA. Fecal weight, colon cancer risk and dietary intake of non-starch polysaccharides (dietary fiber). *Gastroenterology* 1992 ; 103 : 1783-9.
35. Department of Health. *Dietary reference values for food energy and nutrients for the United Kingdom*. Report on Health and Social Subjects. London : HMSO, 1991.

36. WHO. *Diet, nutrition and the prevention of chronic diseases.* Tech Rep Series 797. Geneva : WHO, 1990.
37. Cummings JH. Dietary fibre intakes in Europe : overview and summary of European research activities, conducted by members of the Management Committee of COST 92. In : Carnovale E, Tomassi G, Cumming JH, eds. *Topics in dietary fibre research. Eur J Clin Nutr* 1995 (in press).
38. Burley VJ, Blundell JE. Action of dietary fiber on the satiety cascade. In : Kritchevsky D, Bonfield C, Anderson JW, eds. *Dietary fiber : chemistry, physiology and health effects.* New York : Plenum, 1990 : 227-46.
39. Levine AS, Tallman JR, Grace MK, Parker SA, Billington CJ, Levitt MD. Effect of breakfast cereals on short-term food intake. *Am J Clin Nutr* 1989 ; 50 : 1303-7.
40. de Jong A. Short-chain fatty acids, pancreatic hormones and appetite control. In : Cummings JH, Rombeau JL, Sakata T, eds. *Physiological and clinical aspects of short chain fatty acids.* Cambridge UK : Cambridge University Press, 1995.
41. Anderson JW, Deakins DA, Bridges SR. Soluble fiber ; hypocholesterolemic effects and proposed mechanisms. In : Kritchevsky D, Bonfield C, Anderson JW, eds. *Dietary fiber chemistry, physiology and health effects.* New York : Plenum Press, 1990 : 339-63.
42. Jenkins DJA, Spadafora PJ, Jenkins AL, Rainey-Macdonald CG. Fiber in the treatment of hyperlipidemia. In : Spiller GA, ed. *CRC handbook of dietary fiber in human nutrition*, 2nd edition. Florida : CRC Press, 1993 : 419-38.
43. Thacker PA, Salomons MO, Aherne FX, Milligan LP, Bowland JP. Influence of propionic acid on the cholesterol metabolism of pigs fed hypercholesterolemic diets. *Can J Anim Sci* 1981 ; 61 : 969-75.
44. Chen WL, Anderson JW, Jennings D. Propionate may mediate the hypocholesterolemic effects of certain soluble plant fibers in cholesterol-fed rats. *Proc Soc Exp Biol Med* 1984 ; 175 : 215.
45. Venter CS, Vorster HH, Cummings IH. Effects of dietary propionate on carbohydrate and lipid metabolism in man. *Am J Gastroenterol* 1990 ; 85 : 549-53.
46. Todesco T, Rao AV, Bosello O, Jenkins DJA. Propionate lowers blood glucose and alters lipid metabolism in healthy subjects. *Am J Clin Nutr* 1991 ; 54 : 860-5.
47. Illman RJ, Topping DL, McIntosh GH, *et al.* Hypocholesterolaemic effects of dietary propionate studies in whole animals and perfused rat liver. *Ann Nutr Metab* 1988 ; 32 : 97-107.
48. Vorster HH, Venter CS, Silvis N, van Eeden TS, Huisman HW, Walker ARP. Dietary influences on haemostasis may affect risk for coronary heart disease. *Suid-Afrikaanse Tydskrif vir Wetenskap* 1988 ; 84 : 289-93.
49. Walker ARP, Arvidsson UB. *J Clin Invest* 1954 ; 33 : 1358.
50. Bersohn I, Walker ARP, Higginson J. *S African Med J* 1956 ; 30 : 411.
51. Morris JN, Marr JW, Clayton DG. Diet and heart : a postscript. *Br Med J* 1977 ; 2 : 1307-14.
52. Yano K, Rhoads GK, Kagan A, Tillotson J. Dietary intake and the risk of coronary heart disease in Japanese men living in Hawaii. *Am J Clin Nutr* 1978 ; 31 : 1270-9.
53. Kromhout D, Bosschieter EB, Coulander CL. Dietary fibre and 10-year mortality from coronary heart disease, cancer and all causes. The Zutphen Study. *Lancet* 1982 ; ii : 508-21.
54. Kushi LH, Lew RA, Stare FJ, Ellison CR, Lozy M, Bourke G, Daly L, Graham I, Hickey N, Mulcahy R, Kevaney J. Diet and 20-year mortality from coronary heart disease. The Ireland-Boston Diet-Heart Study. *N Engl J Med* 1985 ; 312 : 811-8.
55. Garcia-Palmieri MR, Sorlie P, Tillotson J, Costas R, Cordero E, Rodriguez M. Relationships of dietary intake to subsequent coronary heart disease incidence : the Puerto Rico Heart Health Program. *Am J Clin Nutr* 1980 ; 33 : 1818-27.
56. Cummings JH, Bingham SA. Towards a recommended intake of dietary fibre. In : Eastwood M, Edwards C, Parry D, eds. *Human nutrition : a continuing debate.* London : Chapman & Hall, 1991 : 107-20.
57. Trowell H. Ischemic heart disease and dietary fiber. *Am J Clin Nutr* 1972 ; 25 : 926-32.

58. Trowell H. Dietary fibre, ischaemic heart disease and diabetes mellitus. *Proc Nutr Soc* 1973 ; 32 : 151-7.
59. Jenkins DJA, Leeds AR, Gassull MA, Wolever TMS, Goff DV, Alberti KGMM, Hockaday TDR. Unabsorbable carbohydrates and diabetes : decreased post-prandial hyperglycaemia. *Lancet* 1976 ; ii : 172-4.
60. British Diabetic Association. Dietary recommendations for diabetics for the 1980's. *Hum Nutr Appl Nutr* 1982 ; 36A : 378-94.
61. Diabetes and Nutrition Study Group of the European Association for the Study of Diabetes. Nutritional recommendations for individuals with diabetes mellitus. *Diabetes Nutr Metab* 1988 ;1 : 145-9.
62. Berger M, Venhaus A. Dietary fibre in the prevention and treatment of diabetes mellitus. In : Schweizer TF, Edwards CA, eds. *Dietary fibre. A component of food.* London : Springer-Verlag, 1992 : 279-93.
63. Wolever TMS, Jenkins DJA. Effect of dietary fiber and foods on carbohydrate metabolism. In : Spiller GA, ed. *CRC handbook of dietary fiber in human nutrition*, 2nd edition. Florida : CRC Press, 1993 : 111-52.
64. Jenkins DJA, Wolever TMS, Leeds AR, Gassull MA, Haisman P, Dilawari J, Goff DV, Metz GL, Alberti KGMM. Dietary fibres, fibre analogues and glucose tolerance : importance of viscosity. *Br Med J* 1978 ; 1 : 1392-4.
65. Kiehm TG, Anderson IW, Ward K. Beneficial effects of a high carbohydrate, high fiber diet on hyperglycemic diabetic men. *Am J Clin Nutr* 1976 ; 29 : 895-9.
66. Crapo PA, Reaven G, Olefsky J. Plasma glucose and insulin responses to orally administered simple and complex carbohydrates. *Diabetes* 1976 ; 25 : 741-7.
67. Crapo PA, Reaven G, Olefsky, J. Postprandial plasma-glucose and insulin responses to different complex carbohydrates. *Diabetes* 1977 ; 26 : 1178.
68. Jenkins DJA, Wolever TMS, Taylor RH, Barker H, Fielden H, Baldwin JM, Bowling AC, Newman HC, Jenkins AL, Goff DV. Glycemic index of foods : a physiological basis for carbohydrate exchange. *Am J Clin Nutr* 1981 ; 34 : 362-6.
69. Asp NG, ed. *Resistant starch.* Proceedings from the 2nd plenary meeting of EURESTA : European FLAIR Concerted Action No. 11 (COST 911) Physiological Implications of the Consumption of Resistant Starch in Man. *Eur J Clin Nutr* 1992 ; 46 : Suppl. 2.
70. Stephen AM. Starch in human nutrition. Symposium Proceedings. *Can J Physiol Pharmacol* 1991 ; 69 : 53-136.
71. Haber GB, Heaton KW, Murphy D, Burroughs LF. Depletion and disruption of dietary fibre : effects on satiety, plasma-glucose and serum insulin. *Lancet* 1977 ; ii : 679-82.
72. Cummings JH. Fermentation in the human large intestine : evidence and implications for health. *Lancet* 1983 ; i : 1206-9.
73. Cummings JH. The effect of dietary fiber on fecal weight and composition. In : Spiller GA, ed. *CRC handbook of dietary fiber in human nutrition*, 2nd edition. Florida : CRC Press, 1993 : 263-349.
74. Cummings JH. Non-starch polysaccharides (dietary fibre) including bulk laxatives in constipation. In : Kamm MA, Lennard-Jones JE, eds. *Constipation.* Petersfield UK : Wrightson Biomedical Publishing Ltd, 1994 : 307-14.
75. Binder HJ, Cummings JH, Soergel KH, *Short chain fatty acids.* Falk Symposium 73. Dordrecht, The Netherlands : Kluwer Academic Publishers, 1994.
76. Cummings JH, Rombeau JL, Sakata T. *Physiological and clinical aspects of short chain fatty acids.* Cambridge, UK : Cambridge University Press, 1995.
77. Roediger WEW. Role of anaerobic bacteria in the metabolic welfare of the colonic mucosa in man. *Gut* 1980 ; 21 : 793-8.
78. Roediger WEW. Utilization of nutrients by isolated epithelial cells of the rat colon. *Gastroenterology* 1982 ; 83 : 424.
79. Jacobs LR, Lupton JR. Effect of dietary fibers on rat large bowel mucosal growth and cell proliferation. *Am J Physiol* 1984 ; 246 : G378-G385.
80. Sakata T, Engelhardt Wv. Stimulatory effect of short chain fatty acids on the epithelial cell proliferation in rat large intestine. *Com Biochem Physiol* 1983 ; 74A : 459-62.

81. Goodlad RA, Lenton W, Ghatei MA, Adrian TE, Bloom SR, Wright NA. Effects of an elemental diet, inert bulk and different types of dietary fibre on the response of the intestinal epithelium to refeeding in the rat and relationship to plasma gastrin, enteroglucagon, and PYY concentrations. *Gut* 1987 ; 28 : 171.
82. Cummings JH. Short chain fatty acids. In : Gibson GR, MacFarlane GT, eds. *Human colonic bacteria : role in nutrition, physiology and pathology.* Florida : CRC Press, 1995 (in press).
83. Englyst HN, Hay S, Macfarlane GT. Polysaccharide breakdown by mixed populations of human faecal bacteria. *FEMS Microbiol Ecol* 1987 ; 95 : 163-71.
84. Weaver GA, Krause JA, Miller TL, Wolin MJ. Cornstarch fermentation by the colonic microbial community yields more butyrate than does cabbage fiber fermentation ; cornstarch fermentation rates correlate negatively with methanogenesis. *Am J Clin Nutr* 1992 ; 55 : 70-7.
85. McBurney MI, Thompson LU. *In vitro* fermentabilities of purified fiber supplements. *J Food Sci* 1989 ; 54 : 347-50.
86. Adiotomre J, Eastwood MA, Edwards CA, Brydon GW. Dietary fiber *in vitro* methods that anticipate nutrition and metabolic activity in humans. *Am J Clin Nutr* 1990 ; 52 : 128-34.
87. Titgemeyer EC, Bourquin LD, Fahey GC, Garleb KA. Fermentability of various fiber sources by human fecal bacteria *in vitro*. *Am J Clin Nutr* 1991 ; 53 : 1418-24.
88. Vince AJ, McNeil NI, Wager JD, Wrong OM. The effect of lactulose, pectin, arabinogalactan and cellulose on the production of organic acids and metabolism of ammonia by intestinal bacteria in a faecal incubation system. *Br J Nutr* 1990 ; 63 : 17-26.
89. Wang X, Gibson GR. Effects of the *in vitro* fermentation of oligofructose and inulin by bacteria growing in the human large intestine. *J Appl Bacteriol* 1993 ; 75 : 373-80.
90. Gibson GR, MacFarlane S, Cummings JH. The fermentability of polysaccharides by mixed human faecal bacteria in relation to their suitability as bulk-forming laxatives. *Letts Appl Microbiol* 1990 ; 11 : 251-4.
91. McBurney MI, Thompson LU. Effect of human faecal inoculum on *in vitro* fermentation variables. *Br J Nutr* 1987 ; 58 : 233-7.

2

Physico-chemical properties of dietary fibre in the foregut

M. EASTWOOD

Gastrointestinal Unit, Western General Hospital, Edinburgh EH4 2XU, UK

Following the ingestion of food, there are a series of complex physical inter-reactions in the upper gastrointestinal tract influenced by the ionic, compositional and pH environment. This chapter examines physico-chemical phenomena used by the food industry which are applicable to events in the post-prandial enteric lumen. The multiple physical phases in the intestinal tract which may affect the rate of absorption from the chyme include *(Table I)*.

The chyme, both lipid or water soluble, will also activate various receptors which control motility. The rate of nutrients flow to the enteric surface and subsequent absorption may also depend upon the luminal macromolecular environment. Adding viscous polysaccharides to carbohydrate meals can reduce postprandial blood glucose concentrations [1]. Wheat and maize but not oats modify glucose absorption rate dependent upon the particle size [2]. This effect was originally explained as a delay in gastric emptying time. There is no relationship between gastric emptying rate and postprandial blood glucose concentrations. Nor do viscous polysaccharides inhibit nutrient access to, and transport across the small intestinal epithelium. Two mechanisms bring nutrients into contact with the epithelium : a) intestinal contractions create turbulence, b) convection currents direct luminal contents from the centre of the lumen to the epithelial surface.

Nutrients diffuse through the thin, relatively unstirred layer of fluid adjacent to the epithelium. Increased luminal content viscosity alters both convection and diffusion of the nutrients across the unstirred layer. The reduction in absorption rate with guar gum may be due to the increased resistance by viscous solutions to the convective flows created by intestinal contractions [3].

Dietary fibre interacts with pancreatic and enteric enzymes and their substrates. Human pancreatic enzyme activity is reduced when incubated with most fibre pressure of the order of 1-3 mPa. Cell walls are composites with an amorphous matrix strengthened by cellulose fibres.

Hydrocolloids

Complex carbohydrates are polyhydroxy polymers with a high affinity for the sorption of water. A mixture of water and soluble carbohydrate molecules is highly structured through numerous hydrogen bonds. The concept of local composition within complex molecules is used to describe the thermodynamic behaviour of aqueous carbohydrate solution within hydrocolloids.

Molecules begin to interact as their concentration increases. Eventually they interact so a nucleous forms and becomes stable or precipitates out. Solubilities vary with the type of solute and solvent and temperature, lactose is the least soluble sugar and fructose is the most soluble. During enteric absorption, water must be absorbed at a rate commensurate with the absorption of solutes so that nutrients do not crystalize or settle out in the intestinal tract. This might happen during malabsorption.

Water soluble polymers, gums, pectins and gelatins can cause agglomeration at low concentrations. Polysaccharides can induce agglomeration in free macromolecules in food emulsion. Macromolecules that do not adsorb on to surfaces of emulsion droplets may possess attractive or repulsive forces. A phenomenon known as depletion flocculation can occur between such macromolecules. An important critical factor in such flocculation is the ionic concentration of the solution between the particles or macromolecules.

Increased salt concentration destabilises emulsions. At a specific salt concentration dependent upon the salt valency (critical flocculation concentration), the emulsion spontaneously flocculates.

Crossed-link systems

Many foods are cross-linked systems, either through chemical covalent bonds or cross-links through molecular entanglement or hydrogen or ionic bond cross-linking. Another cross linkage system is found with rubber elasticity. For this, certain requirements must be satisfied :

— the molecules must exhibit liquid properties,
— long chain molecules with freely rotating links,
— weak secondary forces between the molecules,
— interlocking of the molecules at a few sites to form a three dimensional network.

Physical concepts

Luminal contents

- *Solubilisation*

Complex solutions are a feature of gastro-intestinal tract luminal contents. Such solutions can be described by excess Gibbs energy functions [6, 7] to predict phase changes, water activity, solute activity coefficient and to estimate other physicochemical partial equilibrium properties such as solubilities. If liquid mixtures contain constituents of similar size, shape and chemistry, then the excess Gibbs energy can be described by the 2-suffix Margules equation. More complex equations based on random solution properties assume that the molecules are uniformly distributed throughout the mixture and the intermolecular space is similar to that in pure fluids. There should be no specific interactions between molecules so that the dipole interactions and chemical effects and the distribution and orientation are random. This is not the case in biological systems.

- *Free convection*

Mass transfer can produce density gradients and in turn flow (free convection) which contrasts with the forced convection of stirrers, pumps, etc. [8].

When a salt crystal dissolves, there is diffusion into the surrounding solution so that there is a concentration gradient in the water close to the crystal. The solution flows down the concentration gradient and increases the rate of solute mass transfer. Mass transfer and flow together accelerate dissolution, until free convection decreases as the viscosity or the diffusion coefficient increase.

Local concentrations close to a central molecule differ from the bulk concentrations through competition between the various molecules through interactions with the central molecule [9].

- *The van der Waals potential*

The van der Waals potential acts between surfaces or molecules, through interactions between atoms and molecules which are orientated in such a way that they attract each other.

- *The electrostatic layer potential*

A colloidal particle may acquire a surface charge in an electrolyte solution. The surface charge and the diffuse ion layer surrounding the particle form an electrical double layer whose thickness depends on the ionic strength of the electrolyte. When two identically charged surfaces approach each other, a repulsive force occurs.

Electrostatic repulsion depends on the accumulation of ions between the particles and the solute ionic strength. At very low ionic strength, the double layer thickness is of the order of the particle size. When the attractive interactions cause the particles to attach to one another, flocs or aggregates will be formed. These aggregates are of an open disordered structure. The rheological properties of a flocculated suspension change at a critical volume fraction.

- *Concept of plasticiser* [10]

Plasticisation may occur when a material is incorporated into a polymer increasing workability, flexibility and extensibility. Water is the most important plasticiser, particularly in biological systems changing mobility, rheology and mechanical properties. A true solvent is always a plasticiser but a plasticiser is not always a solvent.

Water is an effective plasticiser of starch and other water compatible food polymers. The presence of water does not mean plasticisation has occurred.

Food ingredients are members of homologous families of completely amorphous or partially crystaline polymers, oligomers and monomers, soluble in and/or plasticised by water. The initial sorbed water fraction is most strongly plasticising and unfreezable or bound. The later sorbed water fraction is freezable, and is free, mobile or loosely bound. Plasticisation leads to increased intermolecular space or free volume, decreases local viscosity and increases mobility. Plasticisation, *e.g.* by water, leads to an increase in mobility in amorphous regions of polymers by increasing free volume and decreasing local viscosity.

Bound water or hindered mobility

Water molecules in a solution are a single physical state with degrees of hindered mobility. Individual water molecules are transiently hydrogen bonded to individual polar sites in the solute.

The traditional concept of bound water suggested discrete free and bound physical states of water (free, loosely bound and tightly bound states) to describe the physical states of water molecules in a solution. The solute specific value of W_g' is the maximum amount of water that can act as a plasticiser or a particular solute, rather than the amount of water that is bound. Adding a few water molecules to an anhydrous solute profoundly changes the visco-elastic properties of the solute through water plasticisation, which increases the free volume and decreases the local viscosity. This has a profound effect on the hindered diffusion of water molecules and produces viscous drag. These less mobile water molecules are pulled along with the solute during flow and are freely exchangeable with all of the water in the solution, *i.e.* the water is not bound.

Water molecules bound to polar groups in polymeric solutes are mobile compared to frozen water, exchanging freely and rapidly with other free or bulk water molecules. The traditional view of the « structuring » effect of solutes on water and of water activity leads to the concept of bound water. This idea is being replaced by a new perspective, the mobilising effect of water acting as a plasticiser.

« Plasticising water » is the non ice portion aqueous component of a water: solute mix. The term bound and free implies that there are two types of water, which can be distinguished chemically or physically (energetically). Plasticising and non plasticising conditions (temperature and time dependent) result from different amounts of water but not different types of water. Free and bound implies two types of water that differ physically (energetically). Plasticising and non plasticising describe two different operational conditions.

Many materials can be characterised as demonstrating an elastic and a viscous response, so called viscoelastic behaviour. If a small strain or stress is applied very rapidly to a viscoelastic material, this will respond elastically. If the stress or strain is applied over a prolonged period, the material will flow with a viscous response. The relaxation time of a substance over time is a measurement, called the Deborah number (De). When De is very large, the system behaves as a solid. When De is very small, it behaves like a liquid. When De is approximately unity, the response is viscoelastic.

The different types of viscous response in a steady shear situation are identified by plots of shear stress against shear rate, or viscosity against shear rate. In the simplest case (Newtonian), the flow curve is a straight line extending through the origin. The slope of the curve is equal to the viscosity. However, most substances do not behave in this manner but as a non-Newtonian system.

Polymeric potentials

Particles in a colloidal suspension may be arranged in varying formats. The structure of a colloidal suspension at rest is a balance between interparticle potential and the Brownian motion of the particles. This is a disorder-order transition state.

The consequences (flocculation or stabilisation) of adding a polymer to a colloidal suspension depend upon the chemistry and molecular weight of the polymer. If a polymer is adsorbed onto the particle surface, one of two things may result. If a polymer molecule adsorbs simultaneously to more than one particle, the polymer will hold the particles together. Such bridging flocculation is the result of strong adsorption, at low polymer concentration, of polymers of high molecular weight. If a particle develops a polymeric layer on its surface, intra particle repulsion will result, so called steric stabilisation. This requires a thick layer, strongly attached to the surface, with high surface coverage.

Micelles

Micelles are colloid-sized clusters of molecules which form in conditions above the critical micelle concentration and above the kraft temperature. Each individual solute molecule is held in an organised solvent cage. An important biological micelle is the detergent micelle of bile acids, triacyl glycerols, cholesterol and di- and mono-acyl glycerols which are found in the upper gastrointestinal tract.

Colloids may be lyophilic (solvent attracting) or lyophobic (solvent repelling), hydrophilic or hydrophobic in water. In the upper gastro-intestinal tract, there are complex lipid/micellar/aqueous/hydrocolloid phases.

Sols

A sol consists of free monomers and small aggregates which coexist within and is intimately dispersed throughout the network. Sols are dispersions of solids in liquids or solids in solids.

Gels [8]

All interiors of cells are gels and most foods with a cellular structure are modified gels. Most food products are multicomponent gels, solids containing 50 % and 90 % water. A gel is a three dimensional polymeric network containing large quantities of solvent (aqueous solution), in a system which has mechanical rigidity.

A gel is a semi-rigid lyophilic sol in which all of the dispersion medium is absorbed by the sol particles. Gels contain two dispersed components or phases, one gives a solid character to the gel and the other is a liquid. A food gel is a continuous and well defined network, embedded in a water based solution phase made up of particles or polymers.

The common factor is a structural coherence which gives mechanical properties, *i.e.* very long stress-relaxation time when the material is deformed. These gels have similar mechanical properties to complex solids or complex fluids, *e.g.* visco elasticity and plasticity.

The sol to gel conversion involves aggregation and growth of particles or macromolecules with periods of very rapid growth in aggregate size. The sol aggregates to a progressively more viscous solution. As cross linkage progresses, the sol fraction diminishes and the solid character becomes greater. Eventually most of the free material becomes involved in a gel network. At a critical degree of aggregation, the gel point is reached when the viscosity changes rapidly to infinity. At this critical gel point, one aggregate molecule exceeds the others in size and subsequently becomes a gel network or gel phase. The residual lower molecular weight materials remain in solution. Polysaccharides readily produce physical association networks through disorder to order transformations. The formation of networks is dependent upon temperature, pH, ionic strength, presence of small particles and specific ions, etc.

Gel networks differ in the strength of connecting cross links and in the flexibility of the units which connect together as well as on the level of network heterogeneity. An important property of a gel is its ability to swell or shrink in an appropriate solvent, dependent upon composition and temperature. The behaviour and properties of gels may be affected by the solvents. The degree and type of swelling with organic liquids may be quite different for those with water. The effect of solvent is described by the percolation theory [11].

Gels contain pores of defined size which can be measured by pressure induced flow. Free molecules diffuse through the gel network. In food, gels are complex, formed from more than one network forming substance and solution and include particles of various types as inert fillers.

Principles of flow in disperse systems [12]

The movement of chyme along the gastrointestinal tract can be regarded as flow in a disperse system, *i.e.* a system defined by the presence of a multiplicity of particles. In general, certain presuppositions are required for such systems:
— that there is a straight tube and that resistance is due only to wall shear stress and no part of the resistance is due to pressure distribution,
— the wall shear stress is constant at each point on the wall surface.

Such an approach does not take account of turbulent flow conditions. During laminar tube flow, fluid elements move rectilinearily without acceleration. There can be intense agitation of fluid flow inside a tube, with resultant effects on boundary or surface layers during the flow. The rate of movement in the centre of the tube is different to that at the boundary layer. The further from the wall, the greater the decrease in fluid velocity. It would not be unexpected if similar differences in flow occurred along the gastrointestinal tract. Flow is not uniform and there is also turbulence. There are a multitude of phases in the gastrointestinal tract ; solid, liquid, colloidal and gas bubble phases as well as hydrophobic and hydrophilic phases.

Rheology

As chyme moves along the gastrointestinal tract, polymer flow and diffusion become important. Suspended rigid particles will affect viscosity and flow through the lumen. Such particles increase the rate of energy dissipation during flow compared to the suspension solvent alone. The suspended particles may be deformable rather than rigid, affected by cooking and ionic strength.

Rheology is the science of deformation and flow of matter under stress [13]. The chemistry and osmolality of the solvent is important to the rheology of dilute solutions. The variables include chemical structure, polymer concentration, mean and range of molecular weight, degree of chain branching, the extent of ionisation (for electrolytes), solution pH, ionic strength and the temperature. Most concentrated solutions of polymers and gels possess viscoelastic properties, *i.e.* their inner structure displays a spectrum of characteristic relaxation or retardation times [14-16].

Rheology of concentration suspensions [17]

Concentrated suspensions often consist of particles in the colloidal size range. The interparticle forces have a pronounced effect on the rheologic behaviour. Material can be characterised by two types of rheological behaviour :
— as a solid showing an elastic behaviour, where the deformation is fully recovered after removal of the applied stress or,
— the material is a liquid having a viscous response when flowing under very small stress.

Physical concepts in absorption

Membranes and diffusion barriers

Thin membranes may define rates of mass transfer on either side of the membrane [18]. These altered rates result from physicochemical interactions between the membrane and the diffusing chemicals. The physical interactions include filtration as different components pass through the membrane at individual rates, largely determined by component size. Transfer across membranes, *e.g.* the unstirred layer of the enteric mucosa, requires pressure, *e.g.* osmotic or electrical potential gradients. A membrane may be permeable to solvent but completely or partially impermeable to solute. Flux equations for membrane transport combine osmotic pressure, membrane diffusion and fluid flow. A concentrated solution at high pressure is forced across a membrane into a dilute solution at low pressure. The membrane may be more permeable to solvent than to solute and so a concentration difference develops. This concentration difference in turn produces an osmotic pressure opposing the flow. The pure solvent has a higher free energy than in solution and will flow from one side to another until the pressure in the solution rises sufficiently to prevent this flow. When the flow ceases, the system is in equilibrium with the osmotic pressure difference giving a measure of concentration. The diffusion of electrolytes across membranes is complex. The electrolyte ionisation, the applied electric field and the electrostatic coupling in multicomponent mixtures are important in addition to the osmotic and pressure differences.

Chemical interactions within membranes initiate a variety of diffusion and chemical reactions. These reactions generate unexpected fluxes that are not proportional to the concentration gradient. These progress backward from a region of low solute concentration into a region of high solute concentration. The chemical effects across membranes involve not only concentration differences but also non linear chemical reactions, *e.g.* facilitated diffusion.

Membrane processes involve both diffusion and reversible chemical reactions and produce highly coupled and selected transport.

This is not the case in living tissues where the fluxes of both sodium and glucose are 100,000 greater than expected and their ratio is about 100 times different from calculations from solubilities. The fluxes may reach a maximum value independent of the concentration differences across the membrane. These fluxes are strongly coupled to other fluxes, the flux of glucose causes a flux of sodium and vice versa. Membrane transport shows many characteristics of enzyme kinetics. Mobile carriers have different diffusion coefficients different from left to right than from right to left.

Absorption

The transport of actively and passively absorbed nutrients across epithelium is affected by the unstirred water layer covering the microvillus membrane [19]. The thickness of the microvillus membrane unstirred water varies with health and disease, intestinal movements and changes in the passive permeability properties of the membrane.

There are three aspects to the unstirred layer :
— the effective thickness,
— the effective surface area,
— the solute diffusion coefficient.

The thickness of the unstirred layer and the effective area may vary along the villus. The presence of mucus or fibre, *e.g.* pectin or guar, in the unstirred layer may alter the viscosity and alter the solute diffusion coefficient. When a solute diffuses through a membrane or is transported, there is a significant concentration gradient across the unstirred layer. Water flow across the membrane reduces the concentration of solute on one side. Conditions within the unstirred layer will be altered if there is a mixture of solutes, one of which is absorbed at a different rate to the others. This may cause an increase in the viscosity of the unstirred layer and increase resistance. The molecules of substances such as guar can interact with enteric mucopolysaccharides and mucosal surface to form a complex three dimensional lattice.

A number of factors may affect the absorption of molecules in the gastrointestinal tract :
— diffusion of molecules from the bulk solution to the intestinal epithelia,
— rate of removal of waters of hydration from complex molecules,

— counter diffusion of solutes away from the intestinal surface,
— orientation of the molecules being absorbed into the appropriate form for absorption. Diffusion of molecules along the epithelial surface to an appropriate absorptive site [20].

The driving force for diffusion of molecules from the bulk solution to the intestinal epithelium is the difference between the bulk concentration C_b and the interfacial concentration C_1. The rate of diffusion can be related to the mass transfer conditions in the bulk solution and the rate of diffusion is dependent upon a variety of factors which include viscosity and agitation.

$$G_d = k_d (T, DAB, \mu, N\ldots\ldots) [C_b - C_1]$$

G_d is the absorption rate, k_d is the mass transfer coefficient,
DAB is the molecular diffusivity of the species A through the solution B,
μ is viscosity and N the rate of agitation.

The coefficient k_d is the function of temperature, bulk diffusivity, solution properties (viscosity, etc.) and the relative speed of absorption [21].

Once molecules arrive at the intestinal surface, they are taken up by receptors and transport mechanisms and broken down to smaller molecular weight materials.

Conclusions

Immense advances in the understanding of events in the upper gastrointestinal tract followed the introduction of the concept of glycaemic index. Such studies have run their course. The elegant measurements and logics of the food technologists should now be introduced into studies designed to explain the physiology of the post-prandial state in the upper gastro-intestinal tract.

References

1. Jenkins DJA, Wolever TMS, Leeds AR, et al. Dietary fibres, fibre analogues and glucose tolerance : importance of viscosity. *Br Med J* 1978 ; 1 : 1392-4.
2. Heaton KW, Marcus SN, Emmett PH, Bolton DH. Particle size of wheat, maize, oat test meals ; effects on plasma glucose and insulin responses and rate of starch digestion *in vitro*. *Am J Clin Nutr* 1988 ; 47 : 675-82.
3. Edwards CA, Johnson IT, Read NW. Do viscous polysaccharides reduce absorption by inhibiting diffusion or convection ? *Eur J Clin Nutr* 1988 ; 42 : 307-12.
4. Schneeman BO, Gallaher D. Effects of dietary fibre on digestive enzyme activity and bile acids in the small intestine. *Proc Soc Exp Biol Med* 1985 ; 180 : 409-14.
5. Ross KD. Estimation of water activity in intermediate moisture foods. *Food Technology* 1975 ; 29 : 26-33.
6. Le Maguer M. Thermodynamics and vapour-liquid equilibria. In : Schwarzberg HG, Hartel RW, eds. *Physical chemistry of foods*. Basic Symposium Series. New York : Marcel Dekker, 1992 : 1-47
7. Elworthy PH, Florence AT, Macfarlane CB. *Solubilisation by surface agents*. London : Chapman and Hall Ltd, 1968.
8. Cussler EL. Diffusion. *Mass transfer in fluid systems*. Cambridge : Cambridge University Press, 1984.

9. Wilson GM. A new expression for the excess free energy of mixing. *J Am Chem Soc* 1964 ; 86 : 127-40.
10. Levine H, Slade L. Glass transitions in food. In : Schwarzberg HG, Hartel RW, eds. *Physical chemistry of foods.* Basic Symposium Series. New York : Marcel Dekker, 1992 : 83-222.
11. Hermansson AM. Gel structure of food biopolymers. In : Blanshard JMV, Mitchell JR, eds. *Food structure, its creation and evaluation.* London : Butterworths, 1988 : 25-40.
12. Molerus O. *Principles of flow in disperse systems.* London : Chapman and Hall, 1993.
13. Warburton B. The rheological characterisation of concentrated solutions and gels of water soluble polymers. In : Finch CA, ed. *Chemistry and technology of water soluble polymers.* New York and London : Plenum Press, 1990 : 1-30.
14. Rockland LB, Stewart GF. *Water activity : influences on food quality.* New York : Academic Press, 1991.
15. Nielsen LE. *Predicting the properties of mixture rules in science and engineering.* New York : Marcel Dekker, 1978.
16. Southgate DAT, Johnston IT, Fenwick GR. *Nutrient availability : chemical and biological aspects.* Cambridge : Royal Society of Chemistry, 1989.
17. Bergstrom L. Rheology of concentrated suspensions. In : Pugh RJ, Bergstrom L, eds. *Surface and colloid chemistry in advanced ceramics processing :* 193-244.
18. Cussler EL. *Diffusion. Mass transfer in fluid systems.* Cambridge : Cambridge University Press, 1984.
19. Read NW. *The relationship between intestinal motility and epithelial transport.* Janssen Research Council, 1986.
20. Eastwood MA, Morris ER. Physical properties of dietary fibre that influence physiological function : a model for polymers along the gastrointestinal tract. *Am J Clin Nutr* 1992 ; 55 : 436-42.
21. Hartel RW. Solid liquid equilibriums crystallisation in foods. In : Schwarzberg HG, Hartel RW, eds. *Physical chemistry of foods.* Basic Symposium Series. New York : Marcel Dekker, 1992 : 47-83.

3

Fermentation of polysaccharides by human colonic anaerobes

A.A. SALYERS

Department of Microbiology, University of Illinois, Urbana, IL 61801, USA

Hundreds of papers have been published on the fermentation of dietary polysaccharides in the colon. No attempt will be made to review them here. Instead, this paper will focus on the holes in the available data base, and assumptions that should be reexamined. Three major assumptions underly virtually all work on the colonic fermentation of polysaccharides. One is that all of the numerically predominant species of colonic bacteria have been cultivated. A second is that the identity of the numerically predominant species is well established. A third is that the species of colonic bacteria responsible for the colonic fermentation of polysaccharides have been identified. Although it is true that the majority of colonic bacteria have been cultivated, there are indications that some bacterial groups may have been missed. Even in the case of the bacteria that were cultivated, there have been disputes about the identity of some of the major species. Finally, despite the fact that considerable progress has been made toward identifying colonic species responsible for polysaccharide fermentation and understanding how polysaccharides are degraded by these bacteria, this information is still far from complete. These gaps in the data base become important when attempts are made to formulate hypotheses about such basic questions as how the activities of colonic bacteria affect their human host and whether it is practical or desirable to alter the composition of the microflora or its fermentation end products.

Composition of the human colonic microflora

Limitations of studies on which current concepts are based

Before saying anything about what types of colonic bacteria are responsible for degrading polysaccharides, it is first necessary to review what is known about the composition of the colonic microflora, because studies of polysaccharide breakdown by colonic bacteria start from this base. Any gaps in this base will affect what can be concluded about which groups of bacteria make the largest contribution to the colonic fermentation. The first systematic studies of the human colonic microflora were published in the mid 1970s [1-3]. Two research groups were responsible for this gargantuan undertaking : the research group headed by Moore and Holdeman at the Virginia Polytechnic Anaerobe Laboratory (Blacksburg, VA) and the research group headed by Finegold and Sutter at the Wadsworth VA Hospital (Los Angeles, CA). These two groups used somewhat different approaches to cultivating and identifying the main species of colonic anaerobes. Finegold and Sutter relied heavily on media and tests originally developed for identification of clinical isolates, whereas the approach of Moore and Holdeman combined features of clinical tests and methods used to cultivate and identify rumen bacteria. Despite their somewhat different approaches, the two groups agreed on the identity of the genera, if not the species, of many of the major groups of colonic bacteria. The genera identified as numerically predominant by both groups are : *Bacteroides*, *Eubacterium*, *Bifidobacterium*, and *Peptostreptococcus*.

It is not surprising, however, that the two groups also disagreed on some assignments. For example, Moore and Holdeman reported that a species they identified as *Fusobacterium prausnitzii* accounted for as much as 5 % of the microflora, whereas Finegold and Sutter did not find this as a numerically predominant species. Similarly, Finegold and Sutter identified as a major microflora component a species they called *Lactobacillus acidophilus*, but which is probably not the same as the species used by the food industry. Moore and Holdeman did not list this as one of the major colonic species.

The problem faced by both groups, which probably explains the differences in findings, was that the identification techniques relied on phenotypic characteristics. At the time these studies were done, this type of identification was not as reliable as it is today, because there had been little experience with the cultivation and identification of anaerobes, especially those that were not common clinical isolates. Subsequent analysis of some of the major colonic genera using DNA-DNA hybridization or 16S rRNA sequencing has clarified the identity of some colonic species, but no attempt has been made to use the much more accurate nucleic acid based methods to enumerate systematically the major species of human colonic bacteria. We used DNA probes to enumerate different species of *Bacteroides* in several different human fecal samples [4, 5]. Our approach bypassed the need for growing the bacteria. The results of our analyses agreed in general with the relative levels of the same species found by Moore and Holdeman. No such approach has ever been used, however, to check systematically the levels of the other major groups of colonic bacteria.

Aside from the uncertain accuracy of the phenotypic tests used for species identification, the early studies had another important limitation. Except for *Bacteroides* spp., there is little information about the plating efficiency of colonic anaerobes, *i.e.* the number of colonies generated when a given number of bacteria are plated. The plating efficiency can be very low in some cases and may be variable. Thus, the number of colonies is not always an accurate indication of the number of bacteria in the original sample. Both Moore and Holdeman and Finegold and Sutter noted a substantial person-to-person variation in the composition of the microflora. The same genera and species were usually found in most people sampled, but the relative levels of different species varied considerably. It is still not clear whether the person-to-person variation was real or merely an indication of the variability inherent in the use of classical enumeration and identification methods. In our DNA probe study we did not detect nearly as much person-to-person variation as reported by the earlier studies, but our study included only a small number of individuals and this could have influenced the amount of variation seen.

Reasons for thinking that some groups of colonic bacteria remain to be identified

If the current list of numerically predominant bacterial genera is complete, it should be possible to account for all known metabolic activities of the colonic microflora by invoking one or more of these genera. Two examples will be used to illustrate that there are activities whose source cannot be explained adequately on the basis of our current knowledge of the colonic microflora. First, nutritional studies have found repeatedly that about half of the cellulose in the human diet is not recovered in the feces [6, 7]. This result suggests that extensive bacterial digestion of cellulose occurs in the colon and that cellulolytic bacteria should be present in high numbers in all people. Nonetheless, attempts to isolate cellulolytic bacteria from human feces have not been successful in identifying the putative cellulolytic population. In one study, cellulolytic bacteria were found in the feces of about one third of the people tested, but even in people who carried cellulolytic isolates the number of bacteria was too low to explain the amount of cellulose digestion observed in nutritional studies [8]. One explanation of these observations is that the main species of cellulolytic bacteria have not yet been cultivated. It is also possible, however, that the cellulolytic species have been cultivated but not identified as cellulolytic because the wrong type of cellulose was used to assess cellulolytic activity. Traditionally, microbiologists have used microcrystalline cellulose to identify cellulolytic bacteria because microcrystalline cellulose is a purified substrate, but microcrystalline cellulose is not degraded appreciably in the human colon [7]. Rather, the type of cellulose degraded in the colon is the amorphous cellulose found in raw and cooked vegetables. If a type of cellulose that more closely approximates the cellulose normally encountered by human colonic bacteria was used to assess cellulolytic activity, some bacteria now thought not to be cellulolytic might be found to have this activity.

A second example of an activity of colonic bacteria that cannot be adequately explained on the basis of current information about the numerically predominant species of colonic bacteria is the high concentration of butyrate in colon contents. The ratio of butyrate to propionate and acetate is about 1:1:4. The high concentrations of acetate and propionate can be explained easily because all of the known major bacterial genera produce acetate as an end product, and some major genera such as Bacteroides produce propionate as well [9]. Also, some fermentation products such as succinate and lactate, which are produced by major groups of colonic bacteria when grown as pure culture, are not detectable in colon contents and are presumably metabolized by other bacteria to acetate and propionate. The origin of the butyrate is more mysterious. According to published descriptions of fermentation products detected when bacteria are grown in laboratory medium, almost none of the well-established numerically major species of colon bacteria produce butyrate, except for a few species of *Eubacterium* [9]. *Fusobacterium prauznitzii* is presumably a butyrate producer because butyrate is one of the products that distinguishes the genus *Fusobacterium*, but the growth of *F. praunitzii* in culture is so poor that it is difficult to be sure what its fermentation products are. Also, as already mentioned, this species has not been found as a major member of the colonic bacterial population by all groups. Another genus that is known to produce butyrate is the genus *Clostridium*, but levels of clostridia in the colon are thought to be relatively low compared to the major populations. If clostridia are responsible for the butyrate observed in colon contents, their metabolic activity must be much higher than one would expect from their numbers. These observations suggest the possibility that some of the butyrate producers have not been cultivated.

Another possible explanation of the origin of the butyrate in human colon contents is that butyrate production may depend on culture conditions. If so, and if conditions used to grow colonic isolates in pure culture do not favor butyrate production, the ability of some of the major genera to produce butyrate could have been underestimated. An indication that this explanation might be correct comes from a recent report that *Bacteroides* spp., which do not produce detectable levels of butyrate when grown in laboratory medium, apparently produce butyrate when growing in the intestine of colonized germfree mice [10]. This interesting finding underscores the fact that we still know relatively little about the metabolism of even the best studied colonic anaerobes.

Polysaccharide-degrading colonic bacteria

Polysaccharide utilization systems of *Bacteroides* spp.

Results of a survey of colonic isolates, which was done in the late 1970s, suggested that *Bacteroides* spp. were the main polysaccharide utilizers in the human colonic microflora [11, 12]. These surveys had two important limitations. First, they were limited to the bacterial groups that could be cultivated. Second, they were limited to the polysaccharides that were commercially available at the time. For example, xyloglucans were not included because they were not available. Since these early surveys, virtually all of the work done on mechanisms of polysaccharide utilization by the major groups of colonic anaerobes has focused on *Bacteroides* spp. [13]. This emphasis has arisen in part from the belief that *Bacteroides* spp. were likely to be the main polysaccharide utilizers in the colonic microflora but has also been strongly influenced by the fact that *Bacteroides* spp. are easy to grow and are genetically manipulable. The only other genus of human colonic bacteria whose polysaccharide utilization mechanisms have been studied in detail is *Clostridium* [14, 15].

Some *Bacteroides* spp. are remarkable for their ability to utilize a variety of dietary and host-derived polysaccharides. Genetic and biochemical studies of the *Bacteroides* polysaccharide utilisation systems has revealed two interesting features of these utilization systems. First, the genes required for polysaccharide utilization are tightly regulated, so that they are only produced when the bacteria are exposed to the polysaccharide. This regulation appears to occur primarily at the transcriptional level [13].

A second interesting feature of the *Bacteroides* polysaccharide utilization systems is that the bacteria do not excrete polysaccharide-degrading enzymes into the extracellular fluid. Rather, they bind the polysaccharide to a receptor complex on their outer membranes and translocate the polysaccharide into the periplasm where the degradative enzymes are located [13, 16]. This type of system allows the bacteria to sequester the products of enzymatic digestion and to prevent them from diffusing away and being captured by other bacteria in the ecosystem. A limitation of this type of polysaccharide import system is that it appears to be adapted to soluble or well-hydrated polysaccharides. Thus, it is not surprising that *Bacteroides* spp. utilize soluble polysaccharides such as starch, arabinogalactan, chondroitin sulfate and pectins, but grow poorly or not at all on insoluble polysaccharides such as xylans and cellulose. This type of cell surface polysaccharide utilization system is not necessarily limited to soluble polysaccharides, however, because cellulolytic *Clostridium* spp. seem to have a similar type of system that consists of a complex of degradative enzymes, substrate binding proteins and probably product binding proteins, which is anchored in the cell membrane [14, 15]. This type of complex is capable of degrading the insoluble substrate cellulose. The reason may be that the clostridia, being gram positive, do not have an outer membrane and thus do not need to translocate the polysaccharide across the outer membrane. The translocation step is the one that is least likely to work well with insoluble polysaccharides.

Results of genetic and biochemical studies of the importance of various polysaccharides as substrates for *Bacteroides* spp. growing in the colon suggest that *Bacteroides* spp. are scavengers that preferentially utilize low abundance soluble polysaccharides [17-20]. It is important to keep in mind that bacteria may not find the most abundant source of carbohydrate attractive as a carbon source, especially if it is poorly utilized. Instead, bacteria may prefer lower abundance carbohydrate sources that are readily utilized. *Bacteroides* spp. appear to exemplify this type of strategy for carbon source acquisition. The fact that *Bacteroides* spp. seem to specialize in soluble polysaccharides, however, raises anew the question of what bacteria are responsible for the extensive digestion of insoluble polysaccharides such as xylan and cellulose that supposedly occurs in the colon.

Other polysaccharide-utilizing colonic anaerobes

The early surveys of colonic bacteria for the ability to utilize polysaccharides revealed that although *Bacteroides* spp. were remarkable for their ability to utilize many different types of polysaccharides, they were not the only bacteria capable of fermenting polysaccharides. Some species of *Bifidobacterium* and *Eubacterium* were also able to utilize polysaccharides [12]. Polysaccharide utilization by these gram positive anaerobes deserves more attention than it has received, especially in view of the fact that some strains of these genera were able to utilize xylan and some *Eubacterium* species are known to produce butyrate as an end product. As already mentioned, *Clostridium* spp. can utilize cellulose and xylans, but since clostridia are generally found in much lower concentrations than the numerically major genera, their contribution to the colonic fermentation of polysaccharides would be expected to be a minor one. By contrast, the gram positive non-sporeforming anaerobes (especially *Eubacterium* and *Bifidobacterium*) could well be important contributors to the colonic fermentation of polysaccharides. An indirect indication that this might be the case comes from a study in which we attempted to determine the source of the major polysaccharidase activities found in a bacterial fraction from human feces [17, 18]. Amylase, α-glucosidase and polygalacturonase were the highest activities in this fraction. Although *Bacteroides* spp. utilize starches and pectins readily, the enzymes in the bacterial fraction appeared not to be *Bacteroides* enzymes. It is not necessarily the case that the contribution of a particular species to the overall utilization of a particular polysaccharide in the colon is proportional to the activity of the enzymes it produces, but the fact that bacterial enzymes not of *Bacteroides* origin were detected in human feces raises the possibility that bacteria other than *Bacteroides* spp. are making an important contribution to polysaccharide digestion in the colon.

The adaptation phenomenon : still a mystery

People who switch from a low fiber diet to a high fiber diet or who begin taking stool softeners that contain high concentrations of soluble polysaccharides frequently experience abdominal discomfort and flatulence for a period after the dietary switch. If they stay on the new diet long enough, these symptoms disappear. This has been called the adaptation phenomenon. If bacterial polysaccharide utilization genes are regulated, as is the case with *Bacteroides* spp., there will be a lag between the time when the bacteria encounter a new polysaccharide source and the time when the bacteria become able to ferment that polysaccharide. This lag is unlikely to contribute much to the adaptation phenomenon, however, because induction of gene expression occurs within hours, whereas the onset of symptoms and their resolution occurs over a period of many days. Another possible explanation for the adaptation phenomenon is that the sudden appearance of high concentrations of readily fermented polysaccharides causes the polysaccharide utilizers to increase their output of gases such as carbon dioxide and hydrogen as well as their output of short chain fatty acids. Normally, at least some of the gases produced by the polysaccharide fermenters are taken up by methanogens, acetogens or sulfate reducers. The balance between gas producers and gas utilizers will ultimately be reestablished, but the adjustment could well take days. This is only a very speculative hypothesis at present, but it is one that should be considered. This hypothesis also brings up the often forgotten fact that different groups of bacteria in the colon are in equilibrium with each other, and this equilibrium could well play an important role in the interaction between the colonic microflora and its human host. Metabolic interactions between different groups of bacteria is a subject that deserves much more attention than it has received to date. Also, groups of different types of bacteria (sometimes called consortia) may be more efficient at fermenting insoluble substrates like xylan and cellulose than single species. That is, the polysaccharide-degrading activity of pure cultures may provide a misleading impression as to which bacteria make the most important contribution to the colonic fermentation. Bacterial interactions have been studied extensively in the case of ruminal bacteria but have received little attention in the case of human colonic bacteria.

References

1. Moore WEC, Holdeman LV. Human fecal flora : the normal flora of 20 Japanese-Hawaiians. *Appl Microbiol* 1974 ; 27 : 961-79.
2. Holdeman LV, Good IJ, Moore WEC. Human fecal flora : variation in bacterial composition within individuals and a possible effect of emotional stress. *Appl Environ Microbiol* 1976 ; 31 : 359-75.
3. Finegold SM, Sutter VL, Mathisen GE. Normal indigenous intestinal flora. In : Hentges D, ed. *The human intestinal microflora in health and disease.* New York : Academic Press, 1983 : 3-32.
4. Kuritza, AP, Salyers AA. Use of species specific DNA hybridization probe for enumerating *Bacteroides vulgatus* in human feces. *Appl Environ Microbiol* 1985 ; 50 : 958-64.

5. Kuritza AP, Shaughnessy P, Salyers AA. Enumeration of polysaccharide degrading *Bacteroides* species in human feces using species-specific DNA probes. *Appl Environ Microbiol* 1986 ; 51 : 385-90.
6. Van Soest PJ. Dietary fibers : their definition and nutritional properties. *Am J Clin Nutr* 1978 ; 31 : S12-S20.
7. Salyers AA, Leedle JAZ. Carbohydrate metabolism in the human colon. In : *The human intestinal flora in health and disease.* New York : Academic Press, 1983 : 129-146.
8. Ehle FR, Robertson JB, Van Soest PJ. Influence of dietary fibers on fermentation in the human large intestine. *J Nutr* 1982 ; 112 : 158-66.
9. Holdeman LV, Cato EP, Moore WEC. *Anaerobe Laboratory Manual*, 4th ed. Anaerobe Laboratory, Virginia Polytechnic Institute and State University, Blacksburg, VA, 1977.
10. Djouzi Z, Andrieu C, Pelenc B, Popot F, Paul F, Monsan P, Szylit O. Degradation of α-glucooligosaccharides by anaerobic bacteria from the human colon, studies *in vitro* and *in vivo* in gnotobiotic rats. Dietary fiber : mechanisms of action in human physiology and metabolism (Nantes, France), Abstract B5, 1994.
11. Salyers AA, Vercellotti J, West S, WiLkins TD. Fermentation of mucin and plant polysaccharides by strains of *Bacteroides* from the human colon. *Appl Environ Microbiol* 1977 ; 33 : 319-22.
12. Salyers AA, West SEH, Vercellotti JR, Wilkins TD. Fermentation of mucins and plant polysaccharides by anaerobic bacteria from the human colon. *Appl Environ Microbiol* 1977 ; 34 : 529-33.
13. Salyers AA, Valentine P, Hwa V. Genetics of polysaccharide utilization pathways of colonic *Bacteroides* species. In : *Genetics and molecular biology of anaerobic bacteria.* New York : Springer-Verlag, 1993 : 505-16.
14. Belaich JP, Belaich A, Gaudin C, Bagnara C. Genes and proteins involved in cellulose degradation by mesophilic clostridia. In : *Genetics and molecular biology of anaerobic bacteria.* New York : Springer-Verlag, 1993 : 407-11.
15. Aubert JP, Beguin P, Millet J. Genes and proteins involved in cellulose and xylan degradation by *Clostridium thermocellum*. In : *Genetics and molecular biology of anaerobic bacteria.* New York : Springer-Verlag, 1993 : 412-22.
16. Tancula E, Feldhaus MJ, Bedzyk LA, Salyers AA. Location and characterization of genes involved in binding of starch to the surface of Bacteroides thetaiotaomicron. *J Bacteriol* 1992 ; 174 : 5609-16.
17. McCarthy R, Salyers AA. Evidence that polygalacturonic acid is not an important substrate for *Bacteroides* species in the colon. *Appl Environ Microbiol* 1986 ; 52 : 9-16.
18. McCarthy RP, Salyers AA. Assessing the possible role of starch as a carbohydrate source for *Bacteroides vulgatus* growing in the human colon. *Appl Environ Microbiol* 1988 ; 54 : 1911-16.
19. Salyers AA, Pajeau M. Competitiveness of different polysaccharide utilization mutants of *Bacteroides* thetaiotaomicron in the intestinal tracts of germfree mice. *Appl Environ Microbiol* 1989 ; 55 : 2572-8.
20. Valentine PJ, Salyers AA. Use of inducible disaccharidases to assess the importance of different carbohydrate sources for *Bacteroides* ovatus growing in the intestinal tracts of germfree mice. *Appl Environ Microbiol* 1992 ; 58 : 2698-700.

4

The production of short-chain fatty acids in the human colon

P.B. MORTENSEN, I. NORDGAARD

University of Copenhagen, Department of Medicine A-2151, Division of Gastroenterology and Hepatology, Rigshospitalet, 9 Blegdamsvej, DK-2100 Copenhagen, Denmark

Bacterial fermentation of carbohydrates occurs as an important digestive principle in plant eating animals and is not always restricted to the large bowel as in humans. In ruminants, the principal fermentation chamber is the modified stomach (foregut fermenters, *e.g.* sheep), whereas herbivorous mammals without a foregut fermentation chamber (hindgut fermenters, *e.g.* elephants) have a voluminous large intestine often with a very large cecum. In contrast, is the colon short and the cecum absent or very small in carnivorous mammals (*e.g.* dog), because the food eaten is sparse in plant polysaccharides. Omnivorous (including man) do not have foregut fermentation chambers and carbohydrates not absorbed in the small intestine are therefore dependent on degradation by bacteria in the large intestine to short-chain fatty acids (SCFAs), which in contrast to carbohydrate, are readily absorbed by the colon to the host organism where it is further metabolized.

Non-starch polysaccharides (NSP or dietary fibre) are broken down by fermentation only, and represent a large proportion of the energy content in many plant foods, because fermentation of plant polysaccharides and the produced SCFAs are an important energy source for the organism. In plant eating animals it may contributes with 60-90 % of energy requirements [1, 2]. In man too, polysaccharides and polypeptides that escape absorption in the small intestine are fermented by anaerobic bacteria in the large intestine to SCFAs. However, colonic SCFA production constitutes only 5-10 % of the energy requirements in healthy subjects with normal small intestinal function [3-5], and is therefore less important for nutrition in man. The salvage of energy in the large intestine is, however, more important in patients with short bowel and other forms of severe malabsorption.

Substrates fermented to short-chain fatty acids

Colonic SCFA production relates to the diet eaten and to the capacity of the small intestine to digest and absorb the diet. Dietary components estimated not to be absorbed in the small intestine from a typical Western diet and therefore fermented by bacterial degradation in the large bowel are shown in *Table I*. Other figures may apply in other parts of the world where dietary contents of starch and non-starch saccharides are main dietary ingredients.

Carbohydrates are considered to be the quantitatively main substrates for colonic SCFA formation. Dietary carbohydrates include mono-, di-, and oligosaccharides, starch, and nonstarch polysaccharides (NSP or dietary fibre). The intake of fibre has been estimated to 15-30 g/day in the Western part of the world [7]. Starch was earlier believed to be completely hydrolysed and absorbed in the small intestine, but recently it was shown that fractions of starch (resistant starch) avoid small intestinal hydrolysis being undegradable by amylase.

Resistant starch

Bond and Levitt [8-10] estimated 10-20 % of starch (wheat flour, beans, potatoes, wheat flour) to be malabsorbed. Evidence for an incomplete absorption of starch also came from intubation studies of the terminal ileum [11, 12], and by studies on ileostomic outputs [13-16].

Starch is a polymer of glucose [17] hydrolysed by pancreatic amylase, which is the only polysaccharide-degrading enzyme secreted in larger amounts in humans. The enzymatic activity is specific for α-glucosidic linkages in starch and amylase does not cleave other types of bindings between monosaccharides in non-starch polysaccharides [13, 18]. Incomplete hydrolysis of certain variants of starch explains why a fraction of starch is not absorbed in the small intestine [19, 20], consequently named resistant starch.

Non-starch polysaccharides (dietary fibre)

Non-starch polysaccharides are, in contrast to starch, not hydrolysed by small intestinal enzymes and pass undegraded into the colonic lumen. Therefore, the amount of dietary fibre reaching the large bowel equals the quantity eaten.

Table I. Substrates available for colonic fermentation in persons consuming Western diets. (From [6].)

Substrate	Amount (g/d)
Non-starch polysaccharides (fibre)	8-18
Resistant starch	8-40
Oligosaccharides	2-8
Unabsorbed sugars	2-10
Dietary proteins	3-9
Pancreatic and gut secretions	4-6
Mucus	2-3
Sloughed epithelial cells	?

Mono- and oligosaccharides

Dietary monosaccharides are absorbed in the small intestine, whereas alcohols (*e.g.* sorbitol and mannitol), and some disaccharides (*e.g.* lactose, in lactose malabsorbers) may resist digestion. Oligosaccharides occur in small quantities in the human diet, but only maltodextrins are digested in the small intestine [21].

The type and amount of carbohydrates malabsorbed to the colon in patients with small intestinal disease has not been fully elucidated, but a wide range of dietary carbohydrates probably pass into the colon and are fermented by the colonic bacteria in patients with malabsorption as *e.g.*, low intestinal disaccharidase activities [22], short bowel, jejunal-ileal by-pass operation, etc. Intestinal secreted glycoproteins in mucus are also degraded by colonic bacteria, estimated to be in the range of 3 to 4 g/day [11].

Polypeptides

Small intestinal digestion of dietary polypeptides is probably incomplete, too. Approx. 10 % of dietary protein has been calculated to reach colonic bacterial fermentation [23, 24], and contribute to the production of SCFAs [19]. Gastrointestinal diseases as malabsorption, protein loosing enteropathy, inflammation, and bleeding may further increase colonic protein degradation [25, 26].

Triglycerides

Dietary fat is mainly long-chain triglycerides hydrolysed by lipases in the small intestine to long-chain fatty acids. Approximately 5 % of dietary fat passes the terminal ileum [27]. Colonic bacteria hydrolyse dietary fat to the long-chain fatty acids, which may be further hydroxylated by bacterial transformation. However, long-chain fatty acids are not metabolized to SCFAs by colonic bacteria, and hence long-chain fatty acids are not absorbed in the colon. Long-chain fatty acids are therefore excreted in faeces in amounts associated with small intestinal malabsorption, in contrast to the negligible amounts of dietary carbohydrates and proteins recovered in faeces from patients where these dietary components are malabsorbed [28].

Hence, the three main nutrients, carbohydrate, protein, and fat all seems to be malabsorbed to some minor extent in the small intestine in healthy individuals. Only carbohydrates and proteins are further degraded to SCFAs in the large intestine. Malabsorption and SCFA production may, however, increase considerably as a consequence of intestinal diseases.

Colonic production of short-chain fatty acids

The colonic capacity to produce SCFAs may be much more pronounced than suggested by the above calculations made on healthy individuals on Western diets. Perfusion studies have shown that the human colon may absorb approximately 500 kcal/day as SCFAs [29] and compensate for carbohydrate malabsorption in patients with small intestinal disease.

Colonic digestion of nutrients and large bowel absorption of calories (as SCFAs) have been studied in short bowel patients with and without a colonic function, *i.e.*

with and without preserved large intestine [28]. In many of the patients, malabsorption approached half of the calories eaten, which is near the limits of where enteral nutrition is possible. A corresponding hyperphagia of more than twice the basal metabolic rate is a common event. Because long-chain fat is absorbed in the small intestine only, contrasted with the absorption of carbohydrates in both the small and large intestine (as mentioned before), differences in absorptive capacities of nutrients were expected in short bowel patients with and without a functioning colon.

Short bowel patients on isocaloric diets and with preserved colonic function increased the calorie absorption by a mean of 465 kcal/day (range : 300-750 kcal/day), as carbohydrate intake was increased from 20 % to 60 % of total calories [28]. This caloric difference was equivalent to 30 % of total energy absorption, which increased from 50 % to 70 %. In other words, dietary changes in favor of the fraction of food that is fermentable, reduced total loss of calories in faeces from around 50 % to 30 % due to the ability of increasing the colonic SCFA production from carbohydrates. Hence, the digestion in these patients had a striking likeness with digestive principles found in hindgut fermenting animals, *e.g.* horse and elephant. Patients with preserved colonic function had low faecal losses of carbohydrates even when intakes were high, whereas faecal excretions of fat paralleled fat intakes *(Table II)*.

Short bowel patients without large bowel function had similar absorptions of calories on high- and low-carbohydrate diets [28], and faecal excretions of both fat and carbohydrates were proportional to dietary intakes *(Table II)*.

Other investigations have indicated an importance of the colonic SCFA production in patients with intestinal diseases or resections. Nightingale *et al.* [30] found the needs for parenteral supply of calories lower in patients with short bowel of equal lengths if colon was preserved. Bond *et al.* [9] showed that an appreciable fraction of carbohydrate (sucrose) was removed during colonic transit in patients with jejunal by-pass, and other authors found absorption of carbohydrates to be significantly higher than absorption of fat in short bowel patients with remaining colon [31]. Royall *et al.* [32] reported that half of an ingested carbohydrate bread

Table II. Faecal excretions of fat, carbohydrate, and nitrogen in short bowel patients with or without colon in continuity. (From [28].)

Patients	Diet	Faecal		
		Fat	Carbohydrate	Nitrogen
		g/day	g/day	g/day
With colon	60 % carbohydrate	46 ± 10	26 ± 4	6 ± 1
	60 % fat	106 ± 9	28 ± 4	6 ± 1
p		0.002	NS	NS
Without colon	60 % carbohydrate	35 ± 6	80 ± 13	9 ± 1
	60 % fat	69 ± 12	42 ± 5	8 ± 1
p		0.01	0.008	NS

meal was malabsorbed in the small intestine and fermented in the large intestine in patients with short bowel. A considerable latent capacity to produce SCFAs was present in healthy individuals ingesting large amounts of lactulose (160 g/day) [33].

Colonic bacteriology and the influence of individual differences

SCFA production is carried out by enzymes produced from a colonic flora of bacteria containing hundreds of different species in total numbers of 10^{11}-10^{12}/g faeces [34]. More than 95 % are anaerobes [35], and generally half of faecal solids from persons consuming Western diets is due to the weight of bacteria [36]. Approximately 70 g/day of carbohydrates are needed for maintenance and growth of the colonic flora [37], equivalent to calculated amounts of carbohydrates avoiding small intestinal absorption in healthy volunteers [3, 15, 38].

The influence of the individual combined flora on the rate and ratios of SCFAs produced in the colon is obviously a matter of interest. However, in comparison with the large differences that may exist as a function of the type of substrate that is fermented, the impact of the individual flora appears to be modest [39, 40].

Polysaccharide fermentation

The production of SCFAs from malabsorbed polysaccharides is initiated by extracellular secreted microbial enzymes hydrolysing the polysaccharides to their monosaccharide constituents [5]. Considerable differences may exist between the hydrolytic activity in plant eating animals and humans. An example is the fermentation of cellulose that hardly takes place in the human colon in contrast to the pronounced degradation in the large intestine of many plant eating animals, where it may account for most of the SCFAs produced and absorbed.

The water solubility of non-starch polysaccharides appears to be a major discriminatory factor for fermentability in man. Soluble fibre are fermented more readily than insoluble fibre, which often are excreted unmetabolized in faeces, creating faecal bulk rather than contributing to SCFA production [41]. However, once the polysaccharides have been broken down to its constituent monosaccharides, the combined human flora possesses the enzymatic capacity to metabolize any monosaccharide to SCFAs [42].

Resistant starch is degraded to glucose, which is taken up by the microorganisms and metabolized to pyruvate by glycolysis [43]. Hemicelluloses are hydrolysed to the various constituent pentose and hexose sugars [44-46], and the major pathway of the pentose utilization seems to involve hexose synthesis *via* the pentose phosphate pathway, before glycolysis to pyruvate [47]. Pyruvate is metabolized to SCFAs, which are the principal end products of fermentation, not further oxidized due to the anaerobic conditions in the colon.

The amount of total SCFAs produced in faecal homogenates from completely fermentable polysaccharides and glucose indicates that equal quantities of SCFAs (approximately 60 w/w %) are produced from equal amounts of starch (resistant and digestible), pectin and glucose [19, 48, 49]. Høverstad [50] estimated that healthy individuals produced SCFAs in amounts of 220-720 mmol/day in agreement with calculated quantities of SCFAs produced by fermentation of the 30-80 g of carbohydrates estimated to arrive from the small intestine [3, 15, 38].

Intestinal concentrations of short-chain fatty acids

The concentrations of SCFAs in the large intestine are high, ranging from about 60 to 150 mmol/l. The three main acids, acetate (C_2), propionate (C_3), and butyrate (C_4), account for 90-95 % of the total SCFAs, with molar ratios of approximately 60 : 25 : 15 [51], whereas isobutyrate, valerate, isovalerate and hexanoate are only present in small amounts. SCFAs are weak acids with pKa values around 4.8, and at the luminal pH in the large bowel 90-99 % of SCFAs are ionized and constitute the predominant anions.

Measurement of SCFA concentrations in different parts of the intestine in animals and humans [52] has shown regional differences. Concentrations are very low in the sterile parts of the upper gut, increasing to measurable amounts around 2-15 mmol/l in terminal ileum [53], which has comparable low counts of bacteria, 10^5-10^6/g [54]. Concentrations of SCFAs increase to high levels in the cecum and right colon, where the bacterial counts increase abruptly. Concentrations may decrease slightly towards the distal parts of the colon and rectum, still being the predominant anions in faeces [52]. In accordance, pH is lowest (5.4-5.9) in the proximal colon and increases distally to 6.6-6.9 [52], suggesting higher rates of fermentation in the cecum and right colon, where substrate availability is more favourable due to the front position in relation to incoming intestinal substrates.

Factors determining the ratios of SCFAs produced from bacterial fermentation are not fully understood. The monosaccharide composition has been shown to be important in incubation studies with faecal batch cultures [42]. The iso-SCFAs (isobutyrate and isovalerate) are produced by protein degradation (together with any of the other SCFAs) and do not origin from carbohydrates, which is explainable from specific SCFAs produced from different aminoacids [25, 26, 55].

The rate of hydrolysis may have a separate role for the ratios of SCFAs produced, as illustrated in studies on the fermentation of different types of digestible and resistant starch. The rate of *in vitro* fermentation of starch was shown to correspond with the rate of small intestinal hydrolysis by amylase *in vitro* [19]. The more resistant starch degraded more slowly by faecal bacteria and produced less butyrate and propionate than digestible starch [19]. Starch resisting small intestinal degradation, and therefore of relevance for cecal fermentation, may thus be associated with a lower butyrate and propionate production than calculated from fermentation studies on digestible starch. Lately it has been suggested that extremely resistant starch may not only resist hydrolysis by amylase, but also resist degradation by the bacterial enzymes in the large intestine, eventually being recovered unmetabolized in faeces and affecting colonic function as an undegradable dietary fibre [56].

Dietary change has shown less effects on SCFA concentrations than might have been anticipated, and unless dietary intake of fermentable carbohydrate is severely restricted (*e.g.*, starvation) faecal concentrations of SCFAs remain remarkably constant in man, while the daily excretion of SCFAs differs as a function of faecal volume. Dietary changes may, however, influence the molar ratios of individual SCFAs produced. The ingestion of large doses of lactulose (160 g/day) increased the percentage of acetate and lactate considerably in faeces at the expense of the other SCFAs, but even though total colonic production of SCFAs obviously increased many-fold, total organic acid (SCFAs + lactate) concentrations were constant. Hence, production of SCFAs is clearly not in direct proportion to luminal concentrations of SCFAs, because concentrations are comparatively constant over a wide range of SCFA production velocities.

In general SCFA excretion (not concentration) rises in conjunction with faecal volumes, including subjects with diarrhoea [57]. Anatomical studies have indicated that the size of the « chamber of fermentation » is of minor importance when it comes to concentrations of SCFAs [58], but probably not in relation to the total amount produced. Comparably high concentrations of SCFAs are found in patients who have had the majority of their colon resected and in patients who are proctocolectomized, but have had a new bacterial reservoir created as an ileo-anal reservoir [59]. Full understanding of the regulatory mechanisms, which normally keep colonic SCFA concentration high and fairly constant, are not yet achieved.

Lactate production in relation to rates of fermentation

Saccharide malabsorption may increase the rates of colonic fermentation to extents where lactate accumulate. In the vast majority of cases, rapid fermentation of malabsorbed saccharides is advantageous for the host in terms of salvaging calories and avoiding osmotic diarrhea induced by the saccharides. Extremely high rates of colonic fermentation are, however, rarely encountered in patients suffering from the syndrome of lactate acidosis, occurring only in patients with severe malabsorption of easily fermentable saccharides. The patients usually have short bowel or jejuno-ileal intestinal by-pass, with episodes of metabolic acidosis with confusion, ataxia and coma. Blood level of D-lactate is increased, while the concentration of L-lactate may stay normal.

A similar syndrome has been indentified in ruminants. The diet of these animals normally contains slowly degradable nonstarch plant polysaccharides (equivalent to dietary fibre), but if fed more rapidly fermentable carbohydrates, such as starch and sugars, rates of fermentation increase resulting in L- and D-lactate accumulation, and fatal D-lactate acidosis may arise [60]. Hindgut fermenters, including man, are usually protected from the incoming of large amounts of sugars and starch in the colon by the digestion and absorption of these substrates in the small bowel. This protection is lost in short bowel patients, where the fermentation of carbohydrates may increase to injurious levels and cause D-lactate acidosis [61].

Colonic lactate accumulation is associated with an extremely rapid bacterial glycolysis to pyruvate and lactate, which occurs more rapidly than the further conversion of lactate to SCFAs. The rate of carbohydrate (polysaccharide) fermentation is usually limited by the process of hydrolysis [61], but the fermentation of simple sugars, disaccharides and the fraction of starch, which is very rapidly digestible (contrasted by resistant starch), is apparently not limited by the rate of hydrolysis, which makes the further conversion of lactate to SCFAs the rate limiting step, resulting in lactate accumulation.

Bacteria are, unlike mammalian cells, able to produce both isomers of lactate, L and D, and the claimed mechanism of D-lactate acidosis has been that the D-isomer accumulates in the organism because it lacks D-lactate dehydrogenase, while L-lactate is metabolized by the well known L-lactate dehydrogenase [62, 63]. A recent study found, however, that D-lactate probably is degraded in the human organism because high concentrations of D-lactate in plasma may vanish rapidly in patients with D-lactate acidosis [61]. Moreover, the organism seems to be protected against an accumulation of D-lactate, as the syndrome of D-lactate acidosis is only rarely seen in patients with short bowel or intestinal by-pass, and is virtually impossible to induce in spite of high faecal concentrations of lactate in healthy individuals ingesting excessive amounts of lactulose. Further studies of two patients with D-lactate acidosis revealed that these patients had a colonic flora with a tenfold increased potential for lactate formation in the presence of rapidly fermentable saccharides [61]. Extremely high concentrations of D- and L-lactate (< 200 mmol/l) may be registered in faeces during attacks of acidosis, which can be induced by large intakes of lactose, but not by large intakes of polysaccharides (starch) or Lactobacilli.

Although not generally acknowledged, D-lactate oxidation in mammals is in fact catalyzed by D-2-hydroxyacid dehydrogenase, a flavoprotein of widespread occurrence within mitochondria, with highest activities in liver and kidney [64-67]. D-lactate, administered as intravenous infusions or ingested, is concordantly eliminated from the blood with a half-life of 20-40 minutes [68, 69].

Increased levels of colonic and faecal lactate are also encountered in patients with ulcerative colitis [70, 71]. In contrast to the DL-lactate of bacterial origin found in patients with saccharide malabsorption, only L-lactate is produced, which originates from the inflammatory process in the mucosa [72]. However, both D- and L-lactate may be found because bacteria rapidly interconvert the two isomers in the colonic contents [61].

In conclusion, the presence of increased concentrations of lactate in the colonic contents or faeces in cases where inflammation is excluded indicates very high rates of bacterial fermentation of carbohydrates. Fermentation of dietary fibre does not usually result in lactate accumulation, which is most often a result of a fermentation of mono- and disaccharides or rapidly hydrolysed polysaccharides (rapid digestible starch, oligoinulins, etc.). Furthermore, lactate is not an end product and will disappear as the carbohydrates are fermented or more slowly degraded, which eliminates lactate accumulation as it degrades to SCFAs.

Local effects of SCFAs in the colon

SCFAs are attributed several local effects in the large bowel, which in the healthy human may attract more attention than the 5-10 % delivery of calories, associated with the oxidation of absorbed SCFAs. The absorption of SCFAs stimulates sodium and water absorption by Na^+/H^+ exchange [29, 73]. SCFAs are metabolized by mucosal cells and butyrate is probably the preferred metabolic energy source for the colonic epithelium and may account for more than 70 % of the oxygen consumed by human colonocytes [74]. A lack of luminal SCFAs and an impaired mucosal metabolism of butyrate has been associated with ulcerative colitis [70,75], and the use of butyrate enemas in distal ulcerative colitis has shown improvement in clinical and endoscopy scores [76, 77]. The lack of fermentable substrate and SCFA production in non-functioning segments of the large intestine is the probable cause of diversion colitis, which has been reversed by treatments with SCFA-containing enemas [78].

A possible role of butyrate has been highlighted in colonic cancerogenesis because of its effect on cell differentiation. Four studies have investigated faecal levels of SCFAs in patients with colonic neoplasia. Vernia et al. [79] compared patients with colorectal cancer, polyps, and healthy controls, but did not found any significant differences, although patients with rectal cancer showed slightly lower levels of propionate and butyrate than those with more proximal cancers. Weaver et al. [80] investigated SCFA distributions in enema samples from a sigmoidoscopy population and found a significantly lower ratio of butyrate and a higher ratio of acetate, in relation to total SCFAs, in colon polyp and cancer patients (evaluated as one group) compared with normal subjects. Faecal concentrations of butyrate were significantly lower in patients with previous colonic adenomas compared with controls in a study made by Kashtan et al. [81], although the difference was not present when the patients were placed on a balanced diet. No differences in faecal concentrations or molar ratios of SCFAs were seen in a study from Clausen et al. [82] comparing healthy subjects and patients with previous colonic adenomas or colonic cancer.

On the other hand, production rates and ratios of SCFAs may be more important than luminal concentrations, because absorption rates, which are the proportion of SCFA offered the mucosal cells, probably parallel production rather than luminal concentrations. Production rates of SCFAs have consequently been measured in a study on faecal homogenates from patients with former colonic adenomas and cancer [82], which reported that production ratios of butyrate were decreased in patients with colonic adenomas and cancer. Production ratios of butyrate from ispagula and wheat bran added to faecal homogenates from these patients were also reduced. Individuals harboring a colonic flora with low butyrate formation, who in addition have a low supply of carbohydrates for colonic fermentation, due to the ingestion of a low-fibre diet or due to a more efficient small intestinal starch absorption, may hypothetically carry an increased risk of colon cancer development.

Starch absorption has indeed been claimed to be more efficient in patients with colonic adenomas compared with controls [83], but fermentation of starch, evaluated by the breath hydrogen excretion, was later reported to be identical in patients with colonic cancer and healthy controls [84].

Investigations on faecal concentrations and *in vitro* production of SCFAs in 20 patients with familial adenomatous polyposis (gene carriers) with and without polyps found no differences in concentrations and ratios of SCFAs, including butyrate [85]. However, patients with polyps produced less butyrate than healthy controls and patients without polyps.

At the present time there is no simple answer to the question of which fibre to be considered optimal in minimizing the risk for colorectal cancer, but different physiological responses to different dietary fibre indicate that more information is required about properties of ingested fibre, such as fermentability and butyrate production.

Systemic effects of SCFAs

SCFAs not metabolized in the mucosa enter the portal vein after absorption [86]. All three major SCFAs are present in portal blood at concentrations several times greater than in peripheral venous blood, indicating that gut is a major source of these acids, but approximately 90 % of butyrate and 10-50 % of propionate is probably metabolized in the colonic mucosa [1]. A pronounced change in molar ratios of the SCFAs occurs between the gut lumen and portal blood, with increasing proportion of acetate, which, unlike butyrate and propionate, in part escapes uptake and metabolism in the gut mucosa and clearance in the liver. Acetate eventually accounts for approximately 90 % of SCFAs in peripheral blood [52]. SCFA concentrations in plasma (approximately 0.06 mmol/l) are roughly one third to one fifth of portal concentrations (0.2-0.3 mmol/l) and around one thousandth of luminal concentrations in the large intestine (60-150 mmol/l) [52].

Interesting differences exist between the SCFAs with even numbers of carbon atoms (acetate and butyrate), and propionate with an odd number of carbon atoms. Butyrate and acetate represent the last steps in the fatty acid beta-oxidation being converted to acetyl CoA, and behave as « lipid-like » substrates. Propionate is converted to propionyl CoA, which is gluconeogenic and hence represents a « glucose-like » substrate. Therefore, acetate, propionate and butyrate may have different impact on the oxidative metabolism in the organism.

Conclusions

SCFA production from dietary fibre is an important colonic function integrated in the physiological events within and outside the large intestine. The pattern of SCFAs produced from carbohydrates differ from the SCFAs produced by bacterial protein degradation. The pattern of SCFAs produced do also differ among different carbohydrates including different fibre.

In vitro faecal homogenate incubations appear to be an useful tool for the initial screening of the intracolonic fermentation of different substrates. *In vitro* studies should not be expected to disclose minor differences between rather similar types of fibre, but major differences in degrees of fermentability (none, intermediate, or complete), rates of fermentability (very rapid with lactate accumulation, rapid without lactate accumulation, intermediate, or slow), and ratios of SCFAs produced (acetate, propionate, butyrate, valerate, hexanoate, isobutyrate, and isovalerate) are exposed by this simple procedure. Rates of ammonia assimilation from peptides and urea may be a further dimension in the characteristics of carbohydrates in association with fermentability.

The main point is that different fibre are fermented to very different degrees, at very different rates, and to different types of SCFAs. The consequences, however, for health and disease remain to be further investigated.

References

1. Bergman EN. Energy contributions of volatile fatty acids from the gastrointestinal tract in various species. *Physiol Rev* 1990 ; 70 : 567-90.
2. Allo A, Oh JH, Longhurst WM, Connolly GE. VFA production in the digestive systems of deer and sheep. *J Wild Manage* 1973 ; 37 : 202-11.

3. McNeil NI. The contribution of the large intestine to energy supplies in man. *Am J Clin Nutr* 1984 ; 39 : 338-42.
4. Royall D, Wolever TMS, Jeejeebhoy KN. Clinical significance of colonic fermentation. *Am J Gastroenterol* 1990 ; 85 : 1307-12.
5. McNeil NI. Nutritional implications of human and mammalian large intestinal function. *Wld Rev Nutr Diet* 1988 ; 85 : 1-42.
6. Cummings JH, Macfarlane GT. The control and consequences of bacterial fermentation in the human colon. *J Appl Bacteriol* 1991 ; 70 : 443-59.
7. Southgate DAT, Bingham S, Robertson J. Dietary fibre in the British diet. *Nature* 1978 ; 274 : 51-2.
8. Bond JH, Levitt MD. Use of pulmonary hydrogen (H_2) measurements to quantitate carbohydrate absorption. Study of partially gastrectomised patients. *J Clin Invest* 1972 ; 51 : 1219-25.
9. Bond JH, Currier BE, Buchwald H, Levitt MD. Colonic conservation of malabsorbed carbohydrate. *Gastroenterology* 1980 ; 78 : 444-7.
10. Anderson IH, Levine AS, Levitt MD. Incomplete absorption of the carbohydrate in all-purpose wheat flour. *N Engl J Med* 1981 ; 304 : 891-2.
11. Stephen AM, Haddad AC, Philips SF. Passage of carbohydrate into the colon. Direct measurement in humans. *Gastroenterology* 1983 ; 85 : 589-95.
12. Flourié B, Leblond A, Florent Ch, Rautureau M, Bissalli A, Rambaud JC. Starch malabsorption and breath gas excretion in healthy humans consuming low- and highstarch diets. *Gastroenterology* 1988 ; 95 : 356-63.
13. Englyst HN, Cummings JH. Digestion of the polysaccharides of some cereal foods in the human small intestine. *Am J Clin Nutr* 1985 : 42 : 778-87.
14. Englyst HN, Cummings JH. Digestion of polysaccharides of potato in the small intestine of man. *Am J Clin Nutr* 1987 ; 45 : 423-31.
15. Wolever TMS, Cohen Z, Thompson LU, Thorne MJ, Jenkins MJA, Prokipchuk EJ, Jenkins DJA. Ileal loss of available carbohydrate in man : comparison of a breath hydrogen method with direct measurement using a human ileostomy model. *Am J Gastroenterol* 1986 ; 81 : 115-22.
16. Chapman RW, Sillery JK, Graham MM, Saunders DR. Absorption of starch by healthy ileostomates : effect of transit time and of carbohydrate load. *Am J Clin Nutr* 1985 ; 41 : 1244-8.
17. Zobel HF. Molecules to granules : a comprehensive starch review. *Starch/Stärke* 1988 ; 40 : 44-50.
18. Sandberg AS, Andersson H, Hallgren B, Hasselblad K, Isaksson B, Hulten L. Experimental model for *in vivo* determination of dietary fibre and its effect on the absorption of nutrients in the small intestine. *Br J Nutr* 1981 ; 45 : 283-94.
19. Nordgaard I, Mortensen PB, Langkilde AM. Small intestinal malabsorption and colonic fermentation of resistant starch and resistant peptides to short-chain fatty acids. *Nutrition* 1995 (in press).
20. Englyst HN, Kingman SM. Classification of dietary starch into categories of specific physiological importance, 1992. MRC Dunn Clinical Nutrition Centre, 100 Tennis Court RD, CB2 1QL, UK.
21. Englyst HN, Hudson GJ, Cummings JH. The fibre/starch overlap : a new look at food carbohydrates. *Eur J Gastroenterol Hepatol* 1993 ; 5 : 569-73.
22. Bond JH, Levitt MD. Fate of soluble carbohydrate in the colon of rats and man. *J Clin Invest* 1976 ; 57 : 1158-64.
23. Gibson JA, Sladen GE, Dawson AM. Protein absorption and ammonia production : the effects of dietary protein and removal of the colon. *Br J Nutr* 1976 ; 35 : 61-5.
24. Vhacko A, Cummings JH. Nitrogen losses from the human small bowel : obligatory losses and the effect of physical form of food. *Gut* 1988 ; 29 : 809-15.
25. Macfarlane GT, Cummings JH, Allison C. Protein degradation by human intestinal bacteria. *J Gen Microbiol* 1986 ; 132 : 1647-56.

26. Mortensen PB, Holtug K, Bonnén H, Clausen MR. The degradation of amino acids, protein, and blood to short-chain fatty acids in colon is prevented by lactulose. *Gastroenterology* 1990 ; 98 : 353-60.
27. Borgström B, Dahlqvist A, Lundh G, Sjövall J. Studies of intestinal digestion and absorption in the human. *J Clin Invest* 1957 ; 36 : 1521-36.
28. Nordgaard I, Hansen BS, Mortensen PB. Colon as a digestive organ in patients with short bowel. *Lancet* 1994 ; 343 : 373-6.
29. Ruppin H, Bar-Meir S, Soergel KH, Wood CM, Schmitt MG. Absorption of short-chain fatty acids by the colon. *Gastroenterology* 1980 ; 78 : 1500-7.
30. Nightingale JMD, Lennard-Jones JE, Gertner DJ, Wood SR, Bartram CI. Colonic preservation reduces need for parenteral therapy, increases incidence of renal stones, but does not change high prevalence of gall stones in patients with short bowel. *Gut* 1992 ; 33 : 1493-7.
31. Messing B, Pigot F, Rongier M, Morin MC, Ndeindoum U, Rambaud JC. Intestinal absorption of free oral hyperalimentation in the very short bowel syndrome. *Gastroenterology* 1991 ; 100 : 1502-8.
32. Royall D, Wolever TMS, Jeejeebhoy KN. Evidence for colonic conservation of malabsorbed carbohydrate in short bowel syndrome. *Am J Gastroenterol* 1992 ; 87 : 751-6.
33. Holtug K, Clausen MR, Hove H, Christiansen J, Mortensen PB. The colon in carbohydrate malabsorption : short chain fatty acids, pH, and osmotic diarrhoea. *Scand J Gastroenterol* 1992 ; 27 : 545-52.
34. Finegold SM, Sutter VL, Sugihara PT, Edler HA, Lehmann SM, Phillips RL. Fecal microbial flora of Seventh Day Adventist populations and control subjects. *Am J Clin Nutr* 1977 ; 30 : 1781-92.
35. Hill MJ, Drasar BS. The normal colonic bacterial flora. *Gut* 1975 ; 16 : 318-23.
36. Stephen AM, Cummings JH. The microbial contribution to human faecal mass. *J Med Microbiol* 1980 ; 13 : 45-56.
37. Smith CJ, Bryant MP. Introduction to metabolic activities of intestinal bacteria. *Am J Clin Nutr* 1979 ; 32 : 149-57.
38. Jenkins DJA, Cuff D, Wolever TMS, Knowland L, Cohen Z, Prokipchuk E. Digestibility of carbohydrate foods in an ileostomate : relationship to dietary fiber, *in vitro* digestibility and glycemic response. *Am J Gastroenterol* 1987 ; 82 : 709-17.
39. Mortensen PB, Hove H, Clausen MR, Holtug K. Fermentation to short-chain fatty acids and lactate in human faecal batch cultures. Intra- and inter-individual variations versus variations caused by changes in fermented saccharides. *Scand J Gastroenterol* 1991 ; 26 : 1285-94.
40. Mortensen PB, Clausen MR, Bonnen H, Hove H, Holtug K. Colonic fermentation of isphaghula, wheat bran, glucose and albumin to short-chain fatty acids and ammonia evaluated *in vitro* in 50 subjects. *JPEN* 1992 ; 16 : 433-9.
41. Mortensen PB, Nordgaard-Andersen I. The dependence of the *in vitro* fermentation of dietary fibre to short-chain fatty acids on the contents of soluble nonstarch polysaccharides. *Scand J Gastroenterol* 1993 ; 28 : 418-22.
42. Mortensen PB, Holtug K, Rasmussen HS. Short chain fatty acid production from mono- and disaccharides in a fecal incubation system : implications for colonic fermentation of dietary fiber. *J Nutr* 1988 ; 118 : 321-5.
43. Baldwin RL, Wood WA, Emery RS. Conversion of glucose-C[14] to propionate by the rumen microbiota. *J Bacteriol* 1963 ; 85 : 1346-9.
44. Howard BH, Jones G, Purdon MR. The pentosanases of some rumen bacteria. *Biochem J* 1960 ; 74 : 173-80.
45. Morrison IM. The rate and products of degradation of xylans by rumen hemicellulases. *Biochem Soc Trans* 1975 ; 3 : 992-4.
46. Wright DE. Pectic enzymes in rumen protozoa. *Arch Biochem Biophys* 1960 ; 86 : 251-4.
47. Pazur JH, Shuey EW, Georgi CE. The conversion of D-xylose into volatile organic acids by rumen bacteria. *Arch Biochem Biophys* 1958 ; 77 : 387-94.
48. Englyst HN, Macfarlane GT. Breakdown of resistant and readily digestible starch by human gut bacteria. *J Sci Food Agric* 1986 ; 37 : 699-706.

49. Macfarlane GT, Englyst HN. Starch utilization by the human large intestinal microflora. *J Appl Bacteriol* 1986 ; 60 : 195-201.
50. Høverstad T. Studies of short-chain fatty acid absorption in man. *Scand J Gastroenterol* 1986 ; 21 : 257-60.
51. Cummings JH. Short-chain fatty acids in the human colon. *Gut* 1981 ; 22 : 763-79.
52. Cummings JH, Pomare EW, Branch WJ, Naylor CPE, Macfarlane GT. Short chain fatty acids in human large intestine, portal, hepatic and venous blood. *Gut* 1987 ; 28 :1221-7.
53. Newton CR, Bennett AN, Billings JA. Ileal short chain fatty acid concentrations after chemically defined diet. *Arch Mal Appar Dig* 1972 ; 61 : 37.
54. Finegold SM, Sutter VL, Boyle JD, Shimada K. The normal flora of ileostomy and transverse colostomy effluents. *J Infect Dis* 1970 ; 122 : 376-81.
55. Rasmussen HS, Holtug K, Mortensen PB. Degradation of amino acids to short-chain fatty acids in humans. *Scand J Gastroenterol* 1988 ; 23 : 178-82.
56. Prynne CJ, Southgate DAT. The effects of a supplement of dietary fibre on faecal excretion by human subjects. *Br J Nutr* 1979 ; 41 : 495-503.
57. Cummings JH, James WPT, Wiggins HS. Role of the colon in ileal resection diarrhoea. *Lancet* 1973 ; i : 344-7.
58. Mortensen PB, Hegnhø J, Rannem T, Rasmussen HS, Holtug K. Short-chain fatty acids in bowel contents after intestinal surgery. *Gastroenterology* 1989 ; 97 : 1090-6.
59. Nordgaard I, Clausen MR, Mortensen PB. Short-chain fatty acids, lactate and ammonia in ileorectal and ileal pouch contents : a model of cecal fermentation. *JPEN* 1993 ; 34 : 324-31.
60. Dunlop RH, Hammond PB. D-lactic acidosis of ruminants. *Ann NY Acad Sci* 1965 ; 119 : 1109-52.
61. Hove H, Mortensen PB. Colonic lactate metabolism and D-lactic acidosis. *Dig Dis Sci* 1995 (in press).
62. Editorial. The colon, the rumen, and D-lactic acidosis. *Lancet* 1990 ; 336 : 599-600.
63. Cross SA, Callaway CW. D-lactic acidosis and selected cerebellar ataxia. *Mayo Clin Proc* 1984 ; 59 : 202-5.
64. Cammack R. Assay, purification and properties of mammalian D-2-hydroxy acid dehydrogenase. *Biochem J* 1969 ; 115 : 55-64.
65. Tubbs PK, Greville GD. The oxidation of D-hydroxy acids in animal tissue. *Biochem J* 1961 ; 81 : 104-14.
66. Tubbs PK. Effects of inhibitors on mitochondrial D-hydroxyacid dehydrogenase. *Biochem J* 1962 ; 82 : 36-42.
67. Brandt RB, Waters MG, Rispler MJ, Kline ES. D- and L-lactate catabolism to CO_2 in rat tissues. *Proc Soc Exp Biol Med* 1984 ; 175 : 328-35.
68. Connor H, Woods HF, Ledingham JGG. Comparison of the kinetics and utilisation of D(-)- and L(+)-sodium lactate in normal man. *Ann Nutr Metab* 1983 ; 27 : 481-7.
69. De Vrese M, Koppenhoefer B, Barth CA. D-lactic acid metabolism after an oral load of DL-lactate. *Clin Nutr* 1990 ; 9 : 23-8.
70. Vernia P, Gnaedinger A, Hauch W, Breuer RI. Organic anions and the diarrhea of inflammatory bowel disease. *Dig Dis Sci* 1988 ; 33 : 1353-8.
71. Vernia P, Caprilli R, Latella G, Barbetti F, Magliocca FM, Cittadini M. Fecal lactate and ulcerative colitis. *Gastroenterology* 1988 ; 95 : 1564-8.
72. Hove H, Holtug H, Jeppesen PB, Mortensen PB. Butyrate absorption and lactate secretion in ulcerative colitis (submitted).
73. Roediger WEW, Moore A. Effect of short-chain fatty acids on sodium absorption in isolated human colon perfused through the vascular bed. *Dig Dis Sci* 1981 ; 26 : 100-6.
74. Roediger WEW. Role of anaerobic bacteria in the metabolic welfare of the colonic mucosa in man. *Gut* 1980 ; 21 : 793-8.
75. Roediger WEW. The colonic epithelium in ulcerative colitis : an energy deficiency disease ? *Lancet* 1980 ; 2 : 712-5.
76. Scheppach W, Sommer H, Kirchner T, Christl SU, Kasper H. Butyrate irrigation for distal ulcerative colitis (Abstr). *Gastroenterology* 1992 ; 102 (suppl) : A 691.

77. Breuer RI, Buto SK, Christ ML, Bean JB, Vernia P, Paoluzi P, Di Paolo MC, Caprilli R. Rectal irrigation with short-chain fatty acids for distal ulcerative colitis. Preliminary report. *Dig Dis Sci* 1991 ; 36 : 185-7.
78. Harig JM, Soergel KH, Komorowski RA, Wood CM. Treatment of diversion colitis with short-chain fatty acids irrigation. *N Engl J Med* 1989 ; 320 : 23-8.
79. Vernia P, Ciarniello P, Cittadini M, Lorenzotti A, Alessandrini A, Caprilli R. Stool pH and SCFA in colorectal cancer and polyps. *Gastroenterology* 1989 ; 96 : A528.
80. Weaver GA, Krause JA, Miller TL, Wolin MJ. Short chain fatty acid distributions of enema samples from a sigmoidoscopy population : an association of high acetate and low butyrate ratios with adenomatous polyps and colon cancer. *Gut* 1988 ; 29 : 1539-43.
81. Kashtan H, Stern HS, Jenkins DJA, Jenkins AL, Thompson W, Hay K, Marcon N, Minkin S, Bruce WR. Colonic fermentation and markers of colorectal-cancer risk. *Am J Clin Nutr* 1992 ; 55 : 723-8.
82. Clausen MR, Bonnen H, Mortensen PB. Colonic fermentation of dietary fibre to short-chain fatty acids in patients with adenomatous polyps and colonic cancer. *Gut* 1991 ; 32 : 923-8.
83. Thornton JR, Dryden A, Kelleher J, Losowsky MS. Superefficient starch absorption - a risk factor for colonic neoplasia ? *Dig Dis Sci* 1987 ; 32 :1088-91.
84. Nordgaard I, Rumessen JJ, Damgaard Nielsen Aa, Gudmand-Høyer E. Absorption of wheat starch in patients resected for left-sided colonic cancer. *Scand J Gastroenterol* 1992 ; 27 : 632-4.
85. Bradburn DM, Mathers JC, Gunn A, Burn J, Chapman PD, Johnston IDA. Colonic fermentation of complex carbohydrates in patients with familial adenomatous polyposis. *Gut* 1993 ; 34 : 630-6.
86. Dankert J, Zijlstra JB, Wolthers BG. Volatile fatty acids in human peripheral and portal blood : quantitative determination by vacuum distillation and gas chromatography. *Clin Chem Acta* 1981 ; 110 : 301-7.

5

Dietary fibre, fermentation and the colon

C.A. EDWARDS

*Department of Human Nutrition, Glasgow University
Yorkhill Hospitals, Glasgow G3 8SJ, UK*

The major effects of dietary fibre occur in the colon. Here each type of dietary fibre interacts with the highly metabolically active bacterial flora, and the colonic mucosa and muscle to produce idiosyncratic results in terms of colonic fermentation products, absorption, motility patterns and stool output. The possible effects in the colon are listed in *Table I*. The actions of an individual fibre source depend to a large extent on its fermentability. The range of fermentability of different types of dietary fibre is great and difficult to predict. Dietary fibres, however, can be roughly divided into those that are rapidly fermented, such as gum arabic and guar gum, those which are more slowly fermented, such as xanthan and karaya, and those which are hardly fermented at all, such as gellan and wheat bran. The least fermentable fibres are the most likely to increase stool output. Dietary fibre which is highly fermentable is unlikely to have much effect on stool output but will affect bacterial fermentation products in the proximal colon and hence colonic and systemic physiology. Obviously the effect of each type of fibre will be determined by dose. A higher intake of ispaghula, for example, had a much greater effect on stool output than a low dose [1]. This may also be true of more rapidly fermentable fibres such as guar. In one study, guar increased stool output [2] in the rat whereas in a second study where a lower dose was used, it had no effect [3]. This effect of dose may be due in part to a stimulation of motility by distension with a large volume of dietary fibre before fermentation is complete. The impact of fermentation in reducing the effect of fibre on stool output is profound, even the stool bulking action of wheat bran is increased if antibiotics are taken [4]. Dietary fibres which are slowly fermented may have a major influence in the distal colon even if they do not increase stool output significantly [3].

Many of the aspects of dietary fibre and bacterial fermentation products are discussed elsewhere in this book. This chapter will concentrate on the effects related to colonic motor function, absorption and stool output.

The human colon

The diversity of the complex carbohydrates that make up dietary fibre is well known and is now taken into account in most studies of dietary fibre. However, the colon is often treated as a single organ and the effects of dietary fibre or bacterial fermentation products in one part of the colon are often extrapolated as probable effects elsewhere in the colon. This extrapolation is often inevitable because of the inaccessibility of most of the colon during *in vivo* studies in man. The conclusions drawn from such studies, however, must be viewed with caution. Since the very reasons which oblige us to extrapolate from one area of the colon to another when studying dietary fibre, also limit the knowledge we have of the normal physiology of each section of the colon. Even when different sections are studied in isolation, as in some *in vitro* studies [5], the lack of background controlling factors (neural, hormonal) and feedback mechanisms between different sections may limit the applicability of the results to normal colonic physiology. In addition, most of the studies in man are carried out under very artificial conditions, often with a tube in the colon passed *per os* or per anus [6, 7] and often after bowel preparation which may disrupt normal colonic functioning. However, it is well established that there are several differences in the physiology of different regions of the colon and these may relate to a difference in the action of different types of dietary fibre.

The proximal and distal colon differ in several fundamental ways. First they have a different neural and blood supply. The colon is innervated with both sympathetic and parasympathetic nerves but the sympathetic nerves dominate maintaining a tonic inhibition of colonic motor activity. The proximal colon is innervated by the vagus and pelvic nerves along with the splanchnic and lumbar sympathetic systems. The distal colon, however, is innervated by only the pelvic nerves and the lumbar sympathetic system. Stimulation of the parasympathetic nerves causes an increase in contractility but the proximal colon contracts rhythmically whereas the distal colon undergoes tonic contraction. The proximal colon is supplied by the superior mesenteric artery and vein and has greater blood flow than the distal colon [8] which is supplied by the inferior mesenteric artery and vein.

The proximal colon acts mainly as a fermentation and absorption chamber whereas the distal colon is more of a storage organ, although it still has an absorption role. The absorption characteristics of the proximal and distal colon are also different. For example, 92 % of chloride dependant sodium transport in the proximal colon

Table I. Possible effects of dietary fibre on the human colon.

1. Increase in stool output
2. Increase in stool frequency
3. Increase in stool water : more fluid consistency
4. Dilution of colonic contents
5. Increase in colonic fermentation
6. Increase in colonic SCFA
7. Decrease in colonic pH
8. Reduction in availability of toxins, bile acids, etc.
9. Reduction in transit time
10. Increase in flatulence

is electroneutral whereas in the distal colon it is mainly amiloride sensitive [9]. The normal physical properties of the luminal contents of the colon also change along its length. Proximal colonic contents are more liquid with a lower pH and very active bacterial metabolism. Under normal circumstances the content of the distal colon is semi-solid and has a more neutral pH [10, 11]. The type of bacterial metabolism also appears to differ along the colon with more protein digestion and methanogenesis [12] occurring in the distal colon. All of these factors may influence the interaction with dietary fibre at any particular site.

Colonic motility

Another major regional difference in the human colon is the predominant motor pattern of each site. These motility patterns are related to the function of each section. Most colonic contractions consist of ring-like contractions of both circular and longitudinal muscle, causing the relaxed areas to bulge out in haustra. The contractions may move forwards, backwards or remain stationary. The proximal colon has mainly retropulsive and mixing movements. The sigmoid or mid colon has a degree of tonic and phasic motor activity and may delay movement of the content and hold it in the descending colon to allow more water absorption. The stimuli for emptying of the proximal colon and propulsion of the contents through the colon is very little understood but the main stimuli seem to be awakening and ingestion of high calorie meals [6, 7, 13, 14]. The relationship of dietary fibre with these motor patterns is probably very complex and is likely to involve the time of day and the site of the colon as well as the type of dietary fibre. There are very few studies which have studied this problem.

There is a paradox in the colon in the relationship between the intensity of colonic motor activity and transit time. In the small intestine, for the most part increased motor activity is related to an increase in the speed at which contents move along the gut. In the colon however, intense motor activity may reflect production of a barrier to flow and a decreased movement of content. In diarrhoea, short spike bursts (SSB), the electrical equivalent to nonpropagating contractions, are virtually absent [15], but in constipation they are very active [16]. On the other hand, if the contractions are propagated aborally, then increased activity may indicate increased propulsion. Thus it is very difficult to predict the action of increased motor activity or motility index unless there is also measurement of the direction of any propagation of the contractions or a measurement of flow. These factors should be considered when interpreting any studies of the effects of dietary fibre or bacterial products on colonic motility as discussed later.

Colonic bacterial flora

Previous chapters have discussed the bacterial populations in the colon and their fermentation of carbohydrate to short chain fatty acids (SCFA; acetic, propionic, butyric and valeric) and gases CO_2, H_2 CH_4 and H_2S. It is perhaps necessary to re-emphasise the diversity of bacterial species and their metabolic capabilities. It is mainly because of the 400 possible bacterial species that person to person variation in fermentation and the relative effects of dietary fibre are so great. As discussed in the chapter by Abigail Salyers we know so little about which bacteria are responsible for which metabolic pathway or products in the colon. Obviously there is still a lot to learn.

When considering the fermentation of dietary fibre by the colonic microflora and the resultant effects on colonic physiology, it is important to remember that some of the enzymes necessary need to be induced. Thus a fibre which is poorly fermented, when first ingested, may have large effects on stool output but, after it has been ingested for a week, may be well fermented and have very little effect on stool output [17]. This adaptation to fibre intake will also influence other actions of dietary fibre. The human gut is very adaptable and will change to maintain the status quo where possible. Short term studies may be misleading if this is not taken into account. Animal studies have suggested that at 4 weeks the gut is still adapting to the influence of dietary fibre [18].

Dietary fibre and stool output

The dietary fibres which have the greatest effects on stool output are in general the least fermentable [19]. These fibres probably act by virtue of their water holding capacity (WHC). The relationship between WHC and stool output is not simple. Dietary fibres with high WHC are usually those which are the most fermentable [20] and are lost before they reach the rectum. There are exceptions such as gellan and ispaghula which have high WHC but resist fermentation [19, 21]. Moreover, one of the most reliable stool bulkers is wheat bran which has a WHC that is as low as the rest of faecal contents on a normal low fibre diet (about 2 g/g ; 19). It appears that the most important factor for a large effect on stool output is simply for the fibre to appear in stool. The effect is then dependent on the amount of fibre present as well as its residual WHC. The effects of fibre are not restricted to increasing output. Dietary fibre also has a role in changing the consistancy of the stool by increasing the water content and the plasticity, and increasing stool frequency. These actions are not mutually dependent on increasing stool output and may be just as important in disease prevention. They may be related to changes in transit time and water absorption but also appear to be related to fermentation. Tomlin and Read [22] found that an increase in stool frequency in man was not related to stool output after ingestion of a range of dietary fibres but appeared to be associated with fermentation *in vitro* using faeces from the same human subjects. In a rat study, stool water was increased by dietary fibres which were slowly fermented and increased faecal SCFA concentration, but which did not increase faecal dry weight [3]. Rapidly fermented fibre had no effect on stool output suggesting that the rate of fermentation is related to the site of SCFA accumulation which in turn is related to stool water. The fermentability of a fibre is related to the time available for fermentation [23]. If propulsion is stimulated before a slowly fermented fibre is metabolised by the colonic flora, fermentation may spread further around the colon. Thus a dietary fibre with high WHC which is slowly fermented may continue to be fermented throughout the colon and increase distal SCFA and stool water *(Table II)*. The relationship between stool SCFA and water is not really clear. The original concept of SCFA increasing stool output by causing an osmotic load [24] was dismissed when it was found that SCFA were so readily absorbed in the human colon [25, 26] and promoted water and electrolyte absorption. SCFA even appear to reverse some of the secretagogue action of enterotoxins. However, the increase in faecal SCFA concentration produced by slowly fermented fibres in the rat study indicates that the absorption of SCFA is not always efficient and there must be some residual osmotic effect. The increase in stool water may also reflect a direct action of SCFA on motility, however, (discussed below) or delaying of total loss of WHC until there is insufficient time to absorb all the released water when fermentation does occur. There may be other mechanisms not yet identified.

The contribution of bacterial cells to faecal mass should not be forgotten [27]. The water content of bacteria is high. However, it is difficult to quantify the bacterial mass in stool and we do not understand which fibres increase bacterial cell yield and which do not.

Dietary fibres which reliably increase stool output may act by more than one mechanism. In a study comparing the action of bran and ispaghula on colonic function in the rat, some interesting differences were identified. Wheat bran and ispaghula are both effective stool bulkers but have different effects on colonic pressure. This caused some concern for the action of ispaghula in diverticular disease where high colonic pressure is implicated in disease aetiology. The measurement of colonic pressure is an indicator of colonic motor activity but usually measured at only one site. As discussed above, interpretation of such simple measurements is difficult. Increased colonic pressure could either indicate a block to flow or propulsion. As ispaghula is such an effective stool bulker, it would be tempting to attribute this increase in pressure to increased propulsion. In a study in humans with diverticular disease who had swallowed a radiotelemetric pressure pill [28], this increase in motor activity appeared to be confined to the proximal colon where retropulsive motor activity is most prominant, in contrast to the distal colon where most diverticula occur. In the rat study [21], animals that had been fed the same diet for 4 weeks supplemented with either ispaghula or wheat bran had very large differences in their colonic contents. Bran fed animals had a large volume of caecal content but very little material in the colon. Ispaghula fed rats however had very full colons. This suggested a difference in the mode of action with bran stimulating propulsion and ispaghula increasing overall flow throughout the colon.

This raises the question of how some dietary fibres promote propulsion or movement of content through the colon. There are several possible mechanisms. First, there is mechanical stimulation. Distension of the colon by increased bulk or by rapid gas production may induce propulsive motility [29]. The edges of the fibre particles may also be involved. It has been shown in dog [30] and man [31] that

Table II. Possible loss of water holding capacity (WHC) and production of short chain fatty acids (SCFA) from dietary fibres of different fermentability.

	Proximal colon	Mid colon	Distal colon	Faeces
Dietary fibre				
Rapidly fermentable	WHC/SCFA	SCFA		No effect
Slowly fermentable	WHC	WHC/SCFA	SCFA	SCFA Increased water
Poorly fermentable	WHC	WHC	WHC/SCFA	WHC/SCFA Increased wet and dry weight

ingestion of plastic or polystyrene particles can produce increases in stool output, water and frequency and a reduction in transit time comparable to that produced by wheat bran. Propagated colonic contractions were induced by polystyrene in the dog which were similar to those seen with dietary fibre [32]. This is presumably caused by increased stimulation of colonic mechanoreceptors and may explain in some part why coarse wheat bran is more effective than finely ground wheat bran [33]. Secondly, fibre may increase colonic flow by chemical simulation. Some dietary fibres increase delivery of bile acids and fatty acids to the colon either by sequestration or binding in the small intestine [34]. If these are released in the colon they may stimulate not only motility [35] but also secretion [36, 37].

Short chain fatty acids, the products of fibre fermentation, have also been shown to influence colonic motility. Their exact role in determining colonic transit time is unclear. Yajima [5] showed in isolated strips of rat colon that propionate and butyrate stimulated contraction. Acetate had no effect and there was no response in the proximal colon. Squires et al. [38] demonstrated an inhibition of colonic contractions in isolated rat colon by mixtures of SCFA at acid pH. Again, interpreting these effects in terms of flow is very difficult as increased contraction could slow transit and less contraction could allow colonic contents to flow more quickly. In vivo studies in man where motility and flow are measured together at different sites in the colon are needed to clarify this.

SCFA have been shown to increase propulsion in the terminal ileum [39] which may be a mechanism for reducing flow back from the colon. Stomach to caecum transit is also accelerated by SCFA [40]. SCFA have been shown to dilate colonic resistance arteries *in vitro* [41]. This may increase absorption from the colon but the interaction of motility and blood flow needs to be explored.

Predicting dietary fibre action on stool output

It is believed that an increase in stool output reduces the risk of disease [42]. It is very difficult, however, to predict the effect of a fibre. To avoid costly feeding trials it would be useful to be able to predict from *in vitro* assays. This would at first seem simple but measurements of water holding capacity can be misleading [20]. An *in vitro* predictive index has been developed from results of a range of dietary fibres tested in man and *in vitro* [19, 43]. This index includes values for WHC after fermentation along with SCFA production. When compared with the stool output observed by each fibre in man and rats [43], it was found that a log *in vitro* index correlated well with results in man but the rat model was better. *In vitro* results do not predict action of a dietary fibre on stool in one individual well [17] but could be used as a screen for predicting effects in a population. The effect of food processing could also be monitored.

Other effects of fermentation of dietary fibre

The effects of SCFA on cell proliferation are discussed elsewhere but the rate of and site of fermentation may determine the action of a dietary fibre on cell proliferation and the distal colon may not respond to fermentable fibre as much as the proximal colon [44]. All the short chain fatty acids have the potential to act as energy sources in the colon and systemically [45], but within the colon, butyrate is thought to be the most important [46]. This along with its promising effects on cell differentiation [47] means that dietary fibres which increase butyrate and especially butyrate in the distal colon, where most disease occurs, are of major interest. Enemas of SCFA have also been used recently in the treatment of inflammatory bowel disease [48]. It is important not to extrapolate too much from *in vitro* studies, however. In a rat study [21], although wheat bran increased butyrate to the greater extent *in vitro*, it had no effect on butyrate in the distal colon *in vivo*. Conversely, ispaghula which was not expected to have an effect did increase distal colonic butyrate [21].

SCFA and other bacterial metabolites may have several other actions in the colon that have not been fully explored. There are potentially toxic effects of metabolites such as secondary bile acids, hydroxy fatty acids, H_2S, phenols and other catabolic products which need to be explored. Bacteria in the colon have been implicated in the aetiology of several colonic diseases and the role of dietary fibre needs to be understood.

pH

After ingestion of rapidly fermentable substrates such as lactulose, colonic pH may fall as low as 5 [11]. Rapidly fermentable fibres may also decrease pH, but this effect will be seen mainly in the proximal colon and may not occur with lower intakes of some dietary fibre sources [3]. If pH does fall it has several important effects including inhibition of 7 α dehydroxylase [49], the enzyme involved in bacterial bile acid metabolism. A low pH will also promote precipitation or sequestration/binding of potentially toxic molecules such as bile and fatty acids [34] and may inhibit NH_3 production and absorption [50, 51]. Acidic pH and SCFA are also potent inhibitors of pathogenic bacteria [52].

Conclusions

Dietary fibre has many important effects in the colon and these are influenced greatly by bacterial fermentation. The exact action of a dietary fibre is very difficult to predict but its fermentability and the likely site or sites of fermentation in the colon must be considered along with the segmental differences in colonic physiology. We do not fully understand the mechanisms by which dietary fibre retains water in the lumen against an osmotic pressure that may be as much as 5 atmospheres [53]. The potential effects of SCFA mean that the products of fermentation of a dietary fibre may be as important as mechanical effects on stool output. It is very difficult to predict bacterial products from fibre structure and chemistry but there are particular substrates which consistently produce more butyrate (starch, wheat bran) or propionate (ispaghula) *in vitro* and in the rat [54]. This must be explored further and future research may help to design a dietary fibre with optimal effects : increasing both stool ouput and distal colonic butyrate, diluting colonic contents and sequestering potential toxins.

References

1. Edwards CA, Bowen J, Brydon WG, Eastwood MA. The effects of ispaghula on rat caecal fermentation and stool output. *Br J Nutr* 1992 ; 68 : 473-82.
2. Davies IR, Brown JC, Livesey G. Energy values and energy balance in rats fed on supplements of guar gum and cellulose. *Br J Nutr* 1991 ; 65 : 415-33.
3. Edwards CA, Eastwood MA. Caecal and faecal short chain fatty acids and stool output in rats fed diets containing non-starch polysaccharides. *Br J Nutr* 1995 (in press).
4. Kurpad AV, Shetty PS. Effects of antimicrobial therapy on faecal bulking. *Gut* 1986 ; 27 : 55-8.
5. Yajima T. Contractile effect of short-chain fatty acids on the isolated colon of the rat. *J Physiol* 1985 ; 368 : 667-78.
6. Christensen J. The response of the colon to eating. *Am J Clin Nutr* 1985 ; 42 : 1025-32.
7. Narducci F, Bassotti G, Gaburri M, Morelli A. 24 hour manometric recording of colonic motor activity in healthy man. *Gut* 1987 ; 28 : 17-25.
8. Grandison AS, Yates J, Shields R. Capillary blood flow in the canine colon and other organs at normal and raised portal pressure. *Gut* 1981 ; 22 : 223-7.
9. Lubke R, Haag K, Berger E, Knauf H, Gerok W. Ion transport in rat proximal colon in vivo. *Am J Physiol* 1986 ; 251 : G132-9.
10. Meldrum SJ, Watson BW, Riddle HL, Bown RL, Sladen GE. pH profile of gut as measured by telemetric capsule. *Br Med J* 1972 ; 2 : 104-6.
11. Bown RL, Gibson JA, Sladen GE, Hicks B, Dawson AW. Effects of lactulose and other laxatives on ileal and colonic pH as measured by a radiotelemetric device. *Gut* 1974 ; 15 : 999-1004.
12. MacFarlane GT, Gibson GR, Cummings JH. Comparison of fermentation reactions in different regions of the human colon. *J Appl Bacteriol* 1992 ; 72 : 57-64.
13. Holdstock DJ, Misiewicz JJ. Factors controlling colonic motility : colonic pressures and transit after meals in patients with total gastrectomy, pernicious anaemia, and duodenal ulcer. *Gut* 1970 ; 11 :100-110.
14. Kumar D, Williams NS, Waldron D, Wingate DL. Prolonged manometric recording of anorectal motor activity in ambulant human subjects : evidence of periodic activity. *Gut* 1989 ; 30 : 1007-11.
15. Bueno L, Fioramonti J, Frexinos J, Ruckebusch Y. Colonic myoelectrical activity in diarrhoea and constipation. *Hepato-gastroenterology* 1980 ; 27 : 281-9.
16. El- Sharkaway TY. Electrical activity of the muscle layers of the canine colon. *J Physiol* 1983 ; 342 : 67-83.
17. Daly J, Tomlin J, Read NW. The effect of feeding xanthan gum on colonic function in man, correlation with *in vitro* determinants of bacterial breakdown. *Br J Nutr* 1993 ; 69 : 897-902.
18. Walter DJ, Eastwood MA, Brydon WG, Elton RA. An experimental design to study colonic fibre fermentation in the rat : duration of feeding. *Br J Nutr* 1986 ; 55 : 465-75.
19. Adiotomre J, Eastwood MA, Edwards CA, Brydon WG. Dietary Fiber : in vitro methods that anticipate nutrition and metabolic activity in humans. *Am J Clin Nutr* 1990 ; 52 : 128-34.
20. McBurney MI, Horvath PJ, Jeraci JL, Van Soest PJ. Effect of *in vitro* fermentation using human faecal inoculum on the water holding capacity of dietary fibre. *Br J Nutr* 1985 ; 53 : 17-24.
21. Edwards CA, Eastwood MA. Comparison of the effects of ispaghula and wheat bran on rat caecal and colonic fermentation. *Gut* 1992 ; 33 : 1229-33.
22. Tomlin J, Read NW. The relationship between bacterial degradation of viscous polysaccharides and stool output in human beings. *Br J Nutr* 1988 ; 60 : 467-75.
23. Van Soest PJ, Jeraci J, Fosse T, Wrick K, Ehle F. Comparative fermentation of fiber in man and animals. In : Wallace CR, Bells L, eds. *Fiber in human and animal nutrition*. Wellington : The Royal Society of New Zealand, 1982 : 75.
24. Forsythe WA, Chenoweth WL, Benninck MR. Laxation and serum cholesterol in rats fed plant fibres. *J Food Sci* 1978 ; 43 : 1470-6.

25. McNeil NI, Cummings JH, James PT. Short chain fatty acid absorption by the human large intestine. *Gut* 1978 ; 19 : 819-22.
26. Binder HJ, Mehta P. Short chain fatty acids stimulate active sodium and chloride transport in the rat distal colon. *Gastroenterology* 1989 ; 96 : 989-96.
27. Stephen AM, Cumrnings JH. The microbial contribution to human faecal mass. *J Med Microbiol* 1980 ; 13 : 45-56.
28. Thornburn HA, Cartcr KB, Goldberg JA, Finlay IG. Does ispaghula husk stimulate the entire colon in diverticular disease. *Gut* 1992 ; 33 : 352-6.
29. Narducci F, Bassoti G, Gaburri M, Solinas A, Fiorucci S, Morelli A. Distension stimulated motor activity of the human transverse descending and sigmoid colon. *Gastroenterology* 1985 ; 88 : 1515-8.
30. Cherbut C, Ruckebusch Y. Modifications de l'électromyogramme du colon chez le chien. *Gastroenterol Clin Biol* 1984 ; 8 : 955-9.
31. Tomlin J, Read NW. Laxative properties of plastic particles. *Br Med J* 1988 ; 297 : 1175-6.
32. Burrows CF, Merntt AM. Influence of alpha cellulose on myoelectric activity of proximal canine colon. *Am J Physiol* 1982 ; 245 : G301-6.
33. Brodribb AJM, Groves C. Effect of bran particle size on stool weight. *Gut* 1978 ; 19 : 60-3.
34. Eastwood MA, Hamilton D. Studies on the adsorption of bile salts to non-absorbed components of the diet. *Biochim Biophys Acta* 1968 ; 152 : 165-75.
35. Kirwan WO, Smith AN, Mitchell WD, Falconer JD, Eastwood MA. Bile acids and colonic motility in the rabbit and the human. *Gut* 1975 ; 16 : 894-900.
36. Mekhjian KS, Phillips SF, Hoffman AF. Colonic secretion of water and electrolyte induced by bile acids : perfusion studies in man. *J Clin Invest* 1971 ; 50 : 1569-71.
37. Ammon HV, Phillips SF. Inhibition of colonic water and electrolyte absorption by fatty acids in man. *Gastroenterology* 1973 ; 65 : 744-9.
38. Squires PE, Rumsey RDE, Edwards CA, Read NW. Effect of short chain fatty acids on contractile activity and fluid flow in rat colon *in vitro*. *Am J Physiol* 1992 ; 261 : G813-7.
39. Kamath PS, Phillips SF, Zinmeister AR. Short chain fatty acids stimulate ileal motility in humans. *Gastroenterology* 1988 ; 95 : 1496-502.
40. Richardson A, Delbridge AT, Brown NJ, Rumsey RDE, Read NW. Short-chain fatty acids in the terminal ileum accelerate stomach to caecum transit time in the rat. *Gut* 1991 : 32 : 266-9.
41. Mortensen FV, Nielsen H, Mulvanney MI, Hessov I. Short chain fatty acids dilate isolated human colonic resistance arteries. *Gut* 1990 ; 31 : 1391-4.
42. Cummings JH, Bingham SA. Towards a recommended intake of dietary fibre. In : Eastwood MA, Edwards CA, Parry D, eds. *Human nutrition. A continuing debate.* London : Chapman Hall 1992 : 107-29.
43. Edwards CA, Adiotomre J, Eastwood, MA. Dietary fibre : the use of *in vitro* and rat models to predict action of stool output in man. *J Sci Food Agri* 1992 ; 59 : 257-60.
44. Edwards CA, Wilson WG, Hanlon L, Eastwood MA. The effect of dietary fibre content of lifelong diet on colonic cell proliferation in the rat. *Gut* 1992 ; 33 : 1076-9.
47. Augeron C, Laboisse CL. Emergence of permanently differentiated cell clones in a human cancer cell line after treatment with sodium butyrate. *Cancer Res* 1984 ; 44 : 3961-9.
48. Breuer RI, Butro SK, Christl ML, Bean J, Vernia P, Paoluzzi P, Di Paolo, MC, Caprilli R. Rectal irrigation with short chain fatty acids for distal ulcerative colitis. *Dig Dis Sci* 1991 ; 36 : 185-7.
49. Thornton JR. High colonic pH promotes colorectal cancer. *Lancet* 1981 ; 11081-3.
50. Swales SD, Tange JD, Wrong OM. The influence of pH bicarbonate and hypertonicity on the absorption of ammonia from the rat intestine. *Clin Sci* 1970 ; 39 : 769-79.
51. Vince A, Killingsley M, Wrong O. Effect of lactulose on ammonia production in a faecal incubation system. *Gastroenterology* 1978 ; 74 : 544-9.

52. Fay JP, Faries RN. The inhibitory action of fatty acids on the growth of *Escherichia coli*. *J Gen Microbiol* 1975 ; 91223-40.
53. Bleakman D, Naftalin RJ. Hypertonic fluid absorption from rabbit descending colon in vitro. *Am J Physiol* 1990 ; 258 : G377-90.
54. Edwards CA, Rowland IR. Bacterial fermentation in the colon and its measurement. In : Schweizer TF, Edwards CA, eds. *Dietary fibre. A component of food*. London : Springer Verlag, 1992 : 119-36.

6

Effects of short-chain fatty acids on gastro-intestinal epithelial cells

T. SAKATA

*Department of Basic Sciences, Ishinomaki Senshu University
Minamisakai Shinmito 1, Ishinomaki 986, Miyagi, Japan*

Dietary fibers resist autoenzymic digestion and enter the hindgut where they are subjected to microbial digestion. Most water-soluble dietary fibers are digested by microbes to produce gases, microbial cell body and short-chain fatty acids (SCFA) such as acetic, propionic, butyric and valeric acids. Many effects of water-soluble dietary fibers are thus due to the SCFA they produce. Among the various effects of SCFA [1], this review focuses on those concerning gastrointestinal epithelial cells.

SCFA as the metabolic fuel for hindgut epithelial cells

Intestinal epithelial cells have two sources of energy substrates : blood and lumen contents. n-butyric acid, and to a lesser extent propionic acid produced in the hindgut lumen, are the main fuels for colonic epithelial cells [2]. The proportional contribution of n-butyrate to total oxygen consumption is 70 % for cell oxidation in vascularly perfused rat colon, and glucose utilization is reduced by more than 50 % in the presence of n-butyrate. Mammalian small intestine does not use n-butyrate as a respiratory fuel, and the contribution of n-butyrate to respiration increases along the length of the colon. The utilization of propionic and n-butyric acid by hindgut epithelial cells results in low levels of these acids in portal blood and virtually null levels in the peripheral artery.

Effect of SCFA on mucosal blood flow

As mucosal blood flow is critical for the function of energy- and oxygen-demanding gut epithelial cells, SCFA effects on mucosal blood flow in the hindgut will be reviewed here.

SCFA increased the blood flow and oxygen supply of autoperfused denervated dog colon [3]. Instillation of an SCFA mixture into human rectum which had received SCFA enemas for 10 to 15 days increased rectal blood flow 1.5- to 5.0-fold [4]. Moreover, acetic, propionic and n-butyric acids produced concentration-dependent relaxation of artery isolated from human ileum or colon, with a minimal effective concentration of 3 mM for individual acid or 1 mM for a mixture of three acids [5].

These results suggest that the effect of SCFA is local and does not require neural reflex. Mechanical removal of endothelium and the addition of indomethacin, propranolol or phentolamine did not alter the relaxing effect of SCFA *in vitro* [5]. Thus, the effect is not mediated by endothelium-derived relaxing factors such as prostaglandins or alpha- or beta-adrenoreceptors. It is very likely that the relaxing effect of SCFA is exerted directly on smooth muscle cells of the artery.

It is unlikely that a decrease in intracellular pH is involved. However, SCFA produced a drop in intracellular calcium, which may be responsible for the relaxing effect [5].

This relaxing effect of SCFA and the resulting increase in blood flow should provide greater oxygen delivery to mucosal cells, which is essential for oxidation and absorption, thereby facilitating removal of SCFA from the mucosal surface. Thus, the effect of SCFA on blood flow may be a mechanism for maintaining the homeostasis of the hindgut lumen.

Effects of SCFA on water and solute absorption from the hindgut

Absorption of water and NaCl is often retarded when conditions such as parenteral nutrition, feeding of a non-residue diet or administration of antibiotics lead to the suppression of SCFA production in the hindgut. Studies indicate that SCFA stimulated NaCl and water absorption as well as bicarbonate secretion *in vivo* in the hindgut [6, 7]. Such effects have also been found in rats suffering from the heat-stable enterotoxin of *Escherichia coli* [8]. However, as interaction between SCFA and Na transports has not been observed in *in vitro* experiments, the effect of SCFA on Na and water absorption may result from osmotic coupling or solvent drug [9].

Clinical trials concerning the *in vivo* effects of SCFA on absorptive functions indicate that net sodium absorption was increased by SCFA in healthy controls, cholera patients with diarrhea and non-cholera patients with watery diarrhea.

SCFA also stimulated the absorption of ammonia from sheep rumen and horse colon [10, 11]. The ionization of SCFA-anions and ammonium ions may be altered by the transfer of protons from ammonium ions to SCFA-anions, making unionized ammonia and SCFA more lipid-soluble than their ionized forms and facilitating their passage across the mucosal barrier. The physiological and clinical significance of these findings is not entirely clear.

Effect of SCFA on gene expression

The effects of SCFA on cultured cells have been studied far more for butyrate than other acids. Butyrate altered the amounts of some proteins, often in correlation with the level of specific mRNA. Proteins characteristic of cell differentiation are often induced by butyrate, and butyrate can reduce the level of several proteins. Butyrate (1 mM) increased brush-border alkaline phosphatase in the LIM 1215 colorectal cancer cell line, while acetate and propionate had only minor effects [12]. These and similar results show that butyrate can induce the expression of differentiation markers in colorectal cancer cells *in vitro*. However, the importance of these *in vitro* effects in the whole animal is not clear [13].

Butyrate induced ectopic synthesis of glycoprotein hormones such as TSH, FSH, LH and hCG [14]. Butyrate also stimulated the transcription of insulin and glucagon genes as well as steady-state levels of mRNAs in the rat islet cell line.

Butyrate increased hormone receptor in cells containing low levels of receptors and decreased it in those with high levels [14]. For example, butyrate increased thyroid hormone receptor in rat hepatoma cells, rat hepatocytes, human skin fibroblasts and C6 rat glioma cells, all of which have low levels, but down-regulated it in pututiary cells which have high levels [14]. Such apparently conflicting effects of SCFA on receptor expression may account for the effect of SCFA on gut epithelial cell proliferation, *i.e.* an inhibitory effect on transformed cells and a stimulatory effect on normal epithelial cells in which mitotic activity is low (as indicated elsewhere in this paper).

The *in vivo* stimulatory effect of SCFA on epithelial cell proliferation in distant segments of the digestive tract requires blood mediation. If SCFA affect gene expression *in vivo* both on hormones and their receptors, there should be an effect on the proliferation of gut epithelial cells.

The effects of butyric acid on gene expression have been attributed to its inhibitory effect on histone deacetylase and the resulting hyperacetylation of histones, which leads to less tight binding to DNA [14]. Such a situation increases the accessibility of DNA to nucleases and other factors that control gene expression.

Effects of SCFA on gastrointestinal epithelial cell division

Effect of SCFA on the proliferation of isolated cells in culture

SCFA inhibit the proliferation of isolated cells, including rumen epithelial cells [15] and colorectal cancer cell lines [13], in a dose-dependent manner. This effect, which is reversible at lower doses but becomes irreversible at higher doses [16, 17], varies among different acids : butyrate > propionate > acetate. Histone hyperacetylation *(see above)* seems to be responsible for this inhibitory effect.

Effect on rumen epithelial cells

Since the rumen is the main digestion site in ruminant farm animals, the effects of SCFA on rumen epithelial cells have been studied intensively. SCFA stimulated mucosal growth of the rumen at weaning, whereas physical factors were responsible for the development of muscle layers [18, 19].

SCFA stimulated the mitosis of rumen epithelial cells in adult sheep [15, 17]. This effect depends on the rate of administration. Rapid administration within 10 seconds was effective, but not continuous infusion into the rumen for 20 hours. Butyric acid had a stronger effect than acetic or propionic acid. However, SCFA inhibited the proliferation and stimulated the postmitotic expression of keratins of rumen epithelial cells in primary culture [15]. Other studies show that the trophic effect of SCFA *in vivo* is mediated by insulin secretion stimulated by SCFA [20]. Insulin stimulated rumen epithelial mitosis *in vivo* [20] and *in vitro* even under the inhibitory action of n-butyric acid [15].

In vitro stimulatory effect of SCFA on normal gut epithelial cell proliferation in monogastric animals

SCFA stimulated epithelial cell proliferation of histologically normal human cecal biopsy specimens [21]. In this study, biopsied specimens were immediately incubated in SCFA-containing medium for 3 hours and subsequently labeled with ^{3}H-thymidine. The intensity of the effect was on the order of butyrate > propionate > acetate. The effect appeared at 10 mM for butyrate and was already saturating at this concentration. In spite of their trophic effect, SCFA did not expand the proliferative zone in the crypt. Similar results have been observed in biopsied specimens of human ascending colon [22] and in short-term culture of pig distal colon (Adachi and Sakata, unpublished results). The latter study used the cryptal cell production rate as a measure of cell proliferation. SCFA increased the fraction of DNA-synthesizing (S-phase) cells and accelerated entrance into mitosis (M-phase), which occurred within 4 hours of culture. It is noteworthy that neither low pH *per se* nor high sodium concentration stimulated colonic cell proliferation [22]. Moreover, pH did not influence the stimulatory effect of SCFA. These results are in agreement with those of Hoshi [23] who found that intracecal instillation of SCFA increased the cecal tissue mass but that the pH of the instillate did not affect cecal tissue mass or enhance SCFA effect.

It is also of interest that Ca salt of butyrate had less stimulatory effect than Na salt [22]. However, the effects of Na-butyrate and ammonium butyrate did not differ, suggesting that SCFA anions are responsible for this trophic effect.

Although these results indicate a local stimulatory effect of SCFA on hindgut epithelial cell proliferation, it would be premature to conclude that this involves a direct effect of SCFA on epithelial cells. The biopsied specimen may have contained some component of mucosal nerve plexus, and entero-endocrine cells and colonic wall can transmit the signal from lumen SCFA through local neural reflex to epithelial cells [24]. It is also uncertain whether the stimulatory effect of SCFA observed in biopsied human cecum is the same as that in rat experiments [25-27] in which the trophic effect of SCFA did not appear before 1 to 3 days and was dose-dependent over a wide range up to 200 mM [28].

Stimulatory effect of hindgut SCFA on gut epithelial cell proliferation *in vivo*

Brief instillation of SCFA into a temporarily isolated segment of rat colon stimulated DNA synthesis and mitosis of the colon (with or without direct contact with SCFA), esophagus, stomach, jejunum and ileum [29]. Surgical bilateral vagotomy or chemical sympathectomy abolished the effect of SCFA. SCFA given into the hindgut increased the crypt-cell production rate of the small and large intestine [25, 28]. Nonfermentable dietary bulk (kaolin) did not stimulate epithelial cell proliferation of the hindgut or influence the stimulatory effect of SCFA [25]. Thus, it would appear that the stimulatory effects of dietary fibers are not due to physical action, such as abrasion or a bulking, but to the SCFA produced from dietary fiber.

The stimulatory effect of SCFA is dose-dependent and varies among acids (acetic < propionic < n-butyric) [28]. The effect appears within 1 to 3 days when a mixture of SCFA [acetic 100, propionic 20 and n-butyric 60 (mM), 3 ml, twice a day] is given intracecally for at least 2 weeks.

Intracolonic or intravenous infusion of SCFA during total parenteral nutrition reduced mucosal atrophy in the jejunum and ileum, *i.e.* smaller losses of mucosal weight, DNA, RNA and protein [30].

Mechanism for the trophic effect of SCFA *in vivo*

It is clear that SCFA themselves, but not bacterial metabolites of SCFA, are responsible for the trophic effect since SCFA infused into the hindgut of germ-free rats showed a trophic effect on the large and small intestine [28]. As the *in vivo* studies cited above used experimental and control solutions of the same pH, it is likely that protonized SCFA or SCFA-anions rather than protons dissociated from SCFA caused the stimulatory effect. The dose-dependency of the effect, despite the same pH for all test solutions, lends further support to this view. Moreover, recent results showing that pH in cecal instillate had no effect on cecal tissue mass, whereas SCFA increased cecal mass [23], also indicate that it is not pH but rather SCFA or their anions that stimulate cell proliferation.

Results in biopsied human cecal or colonic tissue [21, 22] and in short-term culture of pig distal colon have shown that SCFA can stimulate epithelial cell proliferation at the application site. However, this local mechanism cannot account for the effect on distant segments [28-30] not in direct contact with administered SCFA. Recent studies indicated a systemic mediatory mechanism. The afferent transmission of SCFA in hindgut lumen required neural transmission [31], and both sympathetic and parasympathetic nervous systems were involved in the transmission [32]. Efferent transmission did not require mesenteric neural transmission, suggesting either humoral or cellular transmission [33].

Clinical applications

The effects of SCFA on gut epithelial cells noted above led to the clinical applications of SCFA already referred to in this paper.

SCFA enemas seem to ameliorate the histological score or disease activity index of ulcerative colitis [34]. The supply of energy to colonocytes, which is apparently impaired by ulcerative colitis, may be responsible for this effect [35]. It is also noteworthy that butyrate enemas depressed upper crypt-cell proliferation in ulcerative colitis patients, which may reduce the long-term risk of colonic malignancy. Attempts have also been made to use SCFA to accelerate postoperative intestinal adaptation. After intestinal surgery, patients usually receive total parenteral nutrition, which often produces atrophy [36]. In these conditions, intracolonic or intravenous infusion of SCFA can reduce mucosal atrophy in the jejunum and ileum, *i.e.* smaller losses of mucosal weight, DNA, RNA and protein [30]. Moreover, intraluminal infusion of SCFA increased anastomotic bursting pressure and bowel wall tension during the healing of colonic anastomosis in rats [37]. Greater epithelial proliferation may thus produce faster reepithelialization at the anastomosis, reducing the rate of collagen lysis. Increased blood flow by SCFA may also accelerate the healing process.

Perspectives

SCFA affect various functions of gastrointestinal epithelial cells, even in segments distant from the SCFA production site. These effects contribute at least partly to those of fermentable dietary fibers. The divergent effects of SCFA on *in vivo* and *in vitro* systems indicate that due caution should be exercised in interpreting *in vitro* results, especially with respect to clinical implications.

Most of the SCFA effects discussed here are dose-dependent and vary among acids. Accordingly, effects of fermentable fibers can at least partly and should be considered as the result of SCFA microbially produced from these fibers. In this regard, it is clear that the chemical composition of a fiber cannot be a satisfactory predictor of its effect. Methods need to be developed for the evaluation of dietary fiber as a source of SCFA.

The effects of non-SCFA organic acids such as lactic or succinic acids should receive more attention. Indigestible saccharides can be sources of microbial production of non-SCFA organic acids [23]. Succinic acid, but not SCFA, is the determinant pH factor in the cecal contents of rats fed such saccharides. Hoshi [23] has clearly demonstrated that succinic acid, along with SCFA and lumen pH, is an important determinant of cecal motility. Thus, it is advisable not to overlook the production and effects of non-SCFA organic acid in studies of the effects of fermentable fiber.

References

1. Sakata T. Short-chain fatty acids as a physiological signal from gut microbes. In : Chivers DJ, Langer P, eds. *Digestive system in mammals*. Cambridge : Cambridge University Press, 1995 (in press).
2. Roediger WEW. Cellular metabolism of short-chain fatty acids in colonic epithelial cells. In : *Short-chain fatty acids : metabolism and clinical importance*, Columbus : Ross Laboratories, 1990 : 67-71.
3. Kvietys PR, Granger DN. Effect of volatile fatty acids on blood flow and oxygen uptake by the dog colon. *Gastroenterology* 1980 ; 80 : 962-9.

4. Mortensen FV, Hessov I, Birke H, Korsgaard N, Hielsen H. Microcirculatory and trophic effects of short chain fatty acids in the human rectum after Hartmen's procedure. *Br J Surg* 1991 ; 78 : 1208-11.
5. Mortensen FV, Nielsen H, Mulvany MJ, Hessov I. Short chain fatty acids dilate isolated human colonic resistance arteries. *Gut* 1990 ; 31 : 1391-4.
6. Umesaki Y, Yajima T, Tohyama K, Mutai M. Characterization of acetate uptake by the colonic epithelial cells of the rat. *Pflügers Arch* 1978 ; 388 : 205-9.
7. Bugaut M. Occurrence, absorption and metabolism of short chain fatty acids in the digestive tract of mammals. *Comp Biochem Physiol* 1987 ; 86B : 439-72.
8. Ramakrishna BS, Nance SH, Roberts-Thomson IC, Roediger WEW. The effect of enterotoxins and short chain fatty acids on water and electrolyte fluxes in ileal and colonic loops *in vivo* in the rat. *Digestion* 1990 ; 45 : 93-101.
9. Rechkemmer G. *In vitro* studies of short chain fatty acid transport with intact tissue. In : Binder HJ, Cummings J, Sœrgel KH, eds. *Short chain fatty acids*. Dordrecht : Kluwer Academic Publishers, 1994 : 83-92.
10. Bödeker D, Shen J, Kemkowski J, Höller H. Influence of short-chain fatty acids on ammonia absorption across the rumen wall. *Exp Physiol* 1992 ; 77 : 369-76.
11. Bödeker D. Einfluß von kurzkettigen Fettsèuren auf den Ammoniaktransport durch die Colonschleimhaut von Pferden. In the proceeding of « Europaische Konferenz über dei Ernèhrung dei Pferdes », 1993 : 147-9.
12. Whitehead RH, Young GP, Bhathal PS. Effects of short chain fatty acids on a new human colon carcinoma cell line (LIM 1215). *Gut* 1986 ; 27 : 1457-63.
13. Young GP, Gibson PR. Butyrate and the colorectal cancer cell. In : Binder HJ, Cummings J, Sœrgel KH, eds. *Short chain fatty acids*. Dordrecht : Kluwer Academic Publishers, 1994 : 148-60.
14. Kruh J, Defer N, Tichonicky L. Molecular and cellular effects of sodium butyrate. In : Roche AF, ed. *Short-chain fatty acids : metabolism and clinical importance*. Report of the tenth Ross conference on medical research, Columbus OH : Ross Laboratories, 1991 : 45-9.
15. Galfi P, Neogrady S, Sakata T. Effects of volatile fatty acids on the epithelial cell proliferation of the digestive tract and its hormonal mediation. In : Tsuda T, Sasaki Y, Kawashima R, eds. *Physiological aspects of digestion and metabolism in ruminants*. London ; Academic Press, 1990 : 49-59.
16. Ginsburg E, Salamon D, Sreevalsan T, Freese E. Growth inhibition and morphological changes caused by lipophilic acids in mammalian cells. *Proc Natl Acad Sci USA* 1973 : 70 : 2457-61.
17. Sakata T, Yajima T. Influence of short chain fatty acids on the epithelial cell division of digestive tract. *Quart J Exp Physiol* 1984 ; 69 : 639-48.
18. Tamate H, McGilliard AD, Jacobson NL, Getty R. Effect of various diets on the anatomical development of the stomach in the calf. *J Dairy Sci* 1962 ; 45 : 408-20.
19. Tamate H, McGilliard AD, Jacobson NL, Getty R. Effect of various diets on the histological development of the stomach in the calf. *Tohoku J Agr Res* 1964 ; 14 : 171-93.
20. Sakata T, Hikosaka K, Shiomura Y, Tamate H. Stimulatory effect of insulin on ruminal epithelial cell mitosis in adult sheep. *Br J Nutr* 1980 ; 44 : 325-31.
21. Scheppach W, Bartram P, Richter A, Richter F, Liebold H, Dusel G, Hofstetter G, Ruthlein J, Kasper H. Effect of short-chain fatty acids on the human colonic mucosa *in vitro*. *JPEN* 1992 ; 16 : 43-8.
22. Bartram HP, Scheppach W, Schmid H, Hofmann A, Dusel G, Richter F, Richter A, Kasper H. Proliferation of human colonic mucosa as an intermediate biomarker of carcinogenesis : effects of butyrate, ceoxycholate, calcium. *Cancer Res* 1993 ; 53 : 3283-8.
23. Hoshi S. Nutritional and physiological influences of indigestible saccharides on the gastrointestinal tract. Doctoral Thesis, Tohoku University, Sendai, 1994.
24. Yajima T, Sakata T. Influences of short-chain fatty acids on the digestive organs. *Bifidobacteria Microflora* 1987 ; 6 : 7-14.

25. Sakata T. Effects of indigestible dietary bulk and short chain fatty acids on the tissue weight and epithelial cell proliferation rate of the digestive tract in rats. *J Nutr Sci Vitaminol* 1986 ; 32 : 355-62.
26. Kripke SA, Fox AD, Berman JM, et al. Stimulation of intestinal mucosal growth with intracolonic infusion of short chain fatty acids. *JPEN* 1987 ; 13 : 109-16.
27. Kripke SA, Fox AD, Berman JM, et al. Short chain fatty acids and colonic mucosal growth : importance of butyrate. *Clin Nutr* 1989 ; 6 (suppl) : 38.
28. Sakata T. Stimulatory effect of short-chain fatty acids on epithelial cell proliferation in the rat intestine : a possible explanation for trophic effects of fermentable fibre, gut microbes and luminal tropic factors. *Br J Nutr* 1987 ; 58 : 96-103.
29. Sakata T, Engelhardt WV. Stimulatory effect of short-chain fatty acids on the epithelial cell proliferation in rat large intestine. *Comp Biochem Physiol* 1983 ; A47 : 459-62.
30. Koruda MJ, Rolandelli RH, Zimmaro-Bliss D, et al. Parenteral nutrition supplemented with short chain fatty acids : effect on the small bowel mucosa in normal rats. *Am J Clin Nutr* 1990 ; 51 : 685-9.
31. Frankel WL, Zhang W, Singh A, Klurfeld DM, Don S, Sakata T, Modlin I, Rombeau JL. Mediation of the trophic effects of short-chain fatty acids on the rat jejunum and colon. *Gastroenterology* 1994 ; 106 : 375-80.
32. Reilly K, Frankel W, Klurfeld D, Choi D, Rombeau J. The parasympathetic (PSNS) and sympathetic (SNS) nervous system mediate the systemic effects of short chain fatty acids (SCFA) on jejunal structure and function. *Surgical Forum*, 1993, XLIV, 20-2.
33. Sakata T. Stimulatory effect of short-chain fatty acids on epithelial cell proliferation of isolated and denervated jejunal segment of the rat. *Scand J Gastroenterol* 1989 ; 24 : 886-90.
34. Breuer RI, Buto SK, Christ ML, et al. Preliminary report : rectal irrigation with short-chain fatty acids for distal ulcerative colitis. *Dig Dis Sci* 1991 ; 36 : 185-7.
35. Roediger WEW. The imprint of disease on short chain fatty acid metabolism by colonocytes. In : Binder HJ, Cummings J, Sœrgel KH, eds. *Short chain fatty acids*. Dordrecht : Kluwer Academic Publishers, 1994 : 195-205.
36. Levine GM, Deren JJ, Steiger E, Zinno R. Role of oral intake in maintenance of gut mass and disaccharidase activity. *Gastroenterology* 1974 ; 67 : 975-82.
37. Rolandelli RH, Koruda MJ, Settle RG. Effects of intraluminal infusion of short chain fatty acids on the healing of colonic anastomosis in the rat. *Surgery* 1986 ; 100 : 198-203.

7

Dietary fibre and lipid metabolism in humans

T.M.S. WOLEVER

*Department of Nutritional Sciences, 150 College Street,
University of Toronto, Toronto, Ontario, Canada M55 1A8*

It is well established that certain types of dietary fibre and high fibre foods reduce serum cholesterol, with guar gum, pectin, psyllium, oats, dried legumes and barley having been particularly well studied [1]. By lowering serum cholesterol, dietary fibre may have a role to play in reducing the risk for coronary heart disease as originally proposed by Trowell [2]. Indeed, cholesterol lowering is only one potential way that increasing fibre intake may reduce the risk for heart disease, and there is weak evidence that fibre may have beneficial effects on blood clotting, blood pressure, and body weight. Nevertheless, the link between fibre and cholesterol-lowering has not been widely accepted. This may be because many common fibres and high fibre foods, including wheat bran, many fruit and vegetable fibres and cellulose, do not lower serum chotesterol. In addition, the way in which fibre lowers serum cholesterol has not been clear. However, recent studies have improved our understanding of the mechanisms by which dietary fibre influences cholesterol metabolism.

Outline of cholesterol metabolism

The concentration of cholesterol in the blood reflects a balance between the rate of input of cholesterol into the blood and the rate of removal of cholesterol from the blood *(Figure 1)*. Cholesterol may enter the blood either by being absorbed from the intestine or by being synthesized in the liver. Cholesterol may leave the blood by being taken up by peripheral tissues or by the liver. Cholesterol cannot be oxidized, and the only way it can be removed from the body is by being excreted in the stool. Cholesterol reaches the stool *via* the liver which may secrete it into the bile directly, or convert it to bile acids which are secreted into the gut as bile. Bile functions to emulsify dietary lipids and so greatly enhances the absorption of fat, cholesterol and fat soluble vitamins. Most of the cholesterol and bile acids in

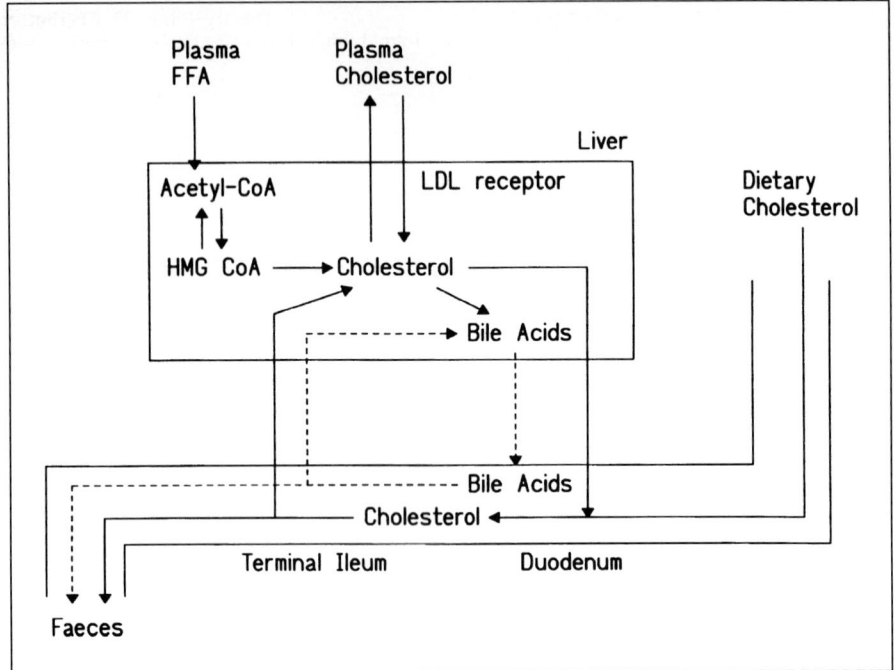

Figure 1. Outline of cholesterol metabolism.

bile are reabsorbed from the gut and undergo an entero-hepatic circulation, with only a small proportion being excreted in the stool. There is evidence that fibre may influence cholesterol metabolism in at least four ways : (1) increased faecal bile acid excretion ; (2) altered absorption of fat and cholesterol ; (3) reduced insulin stimulus to cholesterol synthesis ; and (4) the systemic effects of the short chain fatty acids produced during the fermentation of fibre in the colon *(Figure 2)*. These mechanisms are not mutually exclusive, and may even act in opposite directions in any particular case.

Effect of fibre on lipid metabolism

Increased faecal bile acid excretion

Early studies demonstrated that various types of dietary fibre adsorbed bile acids *in vitro*, increased excretion of bile acids in faeces and altered the spectrum of bile acids excreted [3-5]. Alterations in the ratio of primary to secondary bile acids or an increased excretion of chenodeoxycholic acid and decrease in cholic acid secretion [6] may contribute to the effects of dietary fibre on serum cholesterol. Chenodeoxycholic acid is less well absorbed than cholic acid and may alter hepatic cholesterol synthesis. Thus, changes in the ratio of chenodeoxycholic acid to cholic acid could affect hepatic cholesterol metabolism and serum cholesterol [7]. Increased bile acid excretion has been hypothesized to result in increased cholesterol flux to

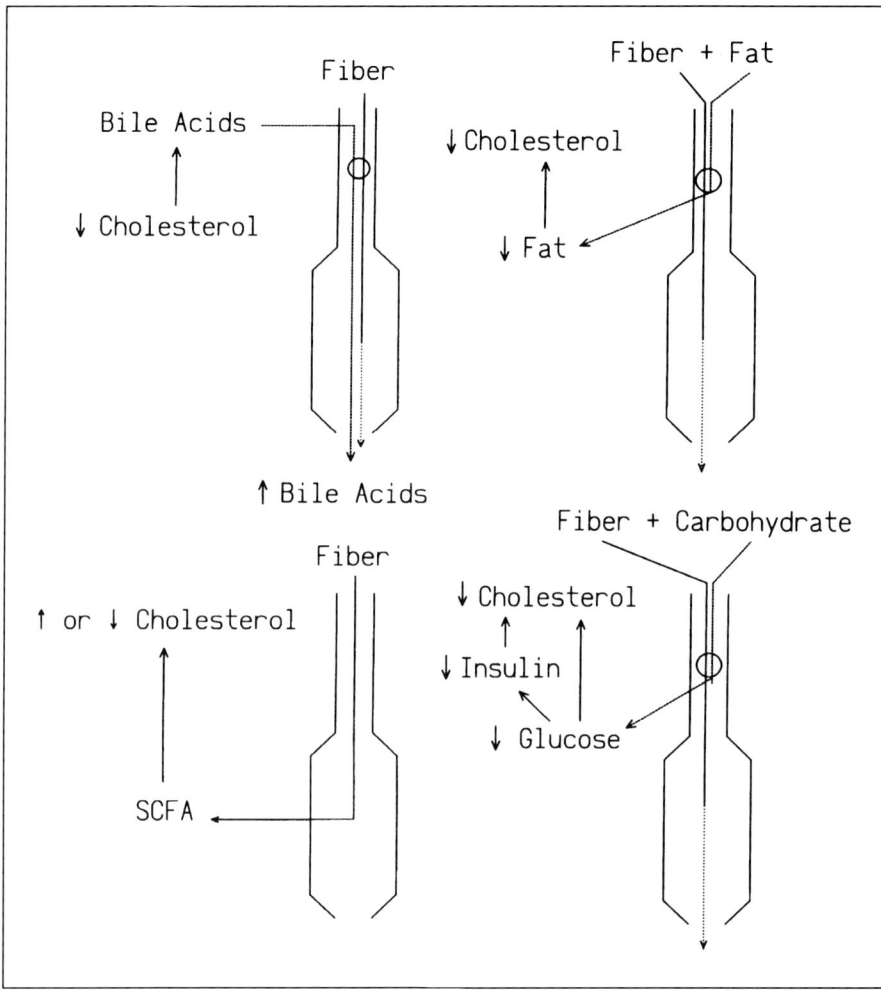

Figure 2. Hypothesized mechanisms by which fibre lowers cholesterol in humans. Upper left : increased faecal bile acid excretion. Upper right : altered lipid absorption. Lower left : effects of colonic short chain fatty acids. Lower right : reduced rate of carbohydrate absorption and reduced stimulus to cholesterol synthesis.

bile acid synthetic pathways with less cholesterol being available for lipoprotein synthetic pathways. For example, 15 g psyllium per day reduced LDL cholesterol in hypercholesterolaemic men, and significantly increased the rate of bile acid synthesis [8].

To see if faecal bile acid excretion was related to the serum cholesterol lowering effect of soluble fibre, we studied 43 mild- to moderately hypercholesterolemic subjects who were given metabolically controlled very low fat diets containing mixed

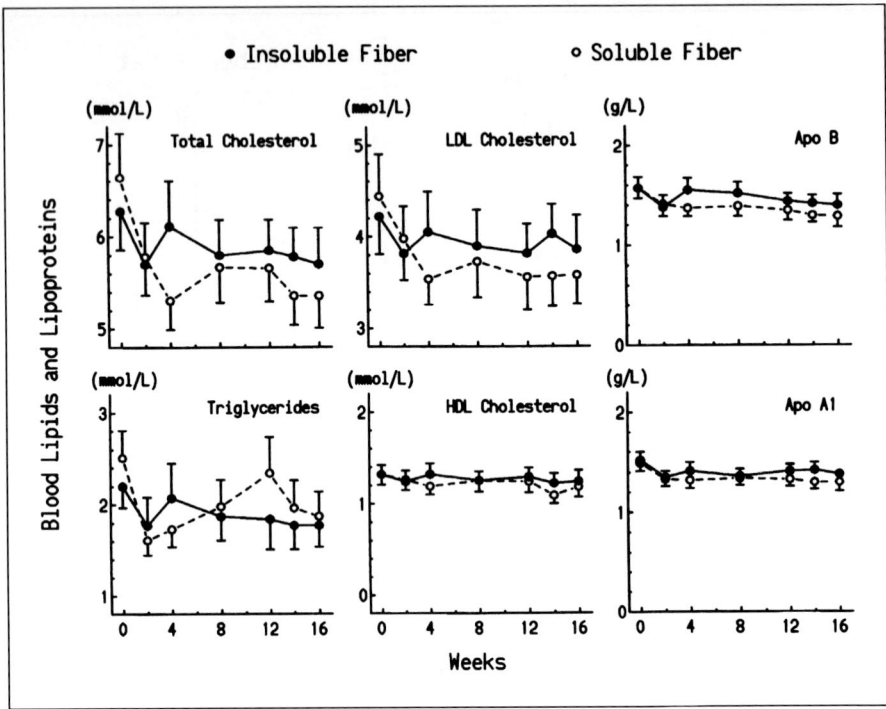

Figure 3. Effect on blood lipids of very high intakes of soluble and insoluble fibre in diets low in saturated fat and cholesterol. Values are means ± SEM for 43 subjects who took metabolic diets for two 16-week periods. (Redrawn from [9].)

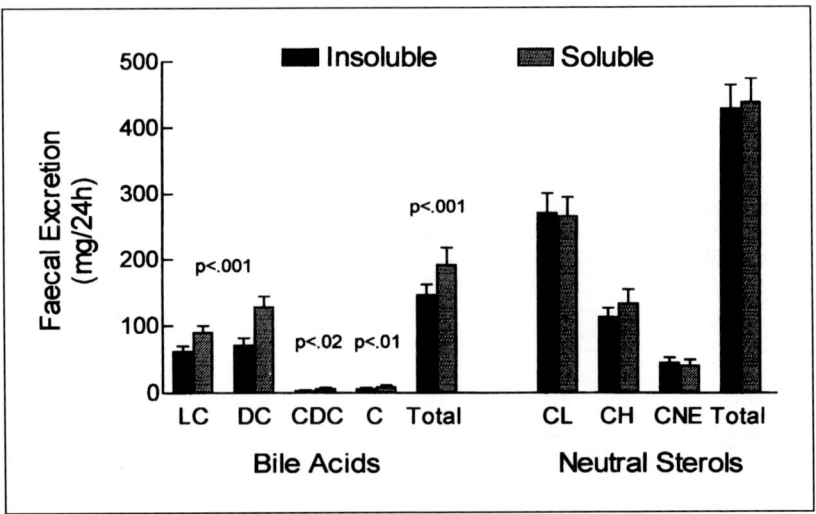

Figure 4. Effect on faecal bile acid and neutral sterol excretion after 15 weeks on diets very high in soluble and insoluble fibre and low in saturated fat and cholesterol. Values are means ± SEM for 42 subjects who took metabolic diets for two 16-week periods. LC denotes lithocolic acid, DC deoxycholic acid, CDC chenodeoxycholic acid, C cholic acid, CL coprostanol, CH cholesterol, and CNE coprostanone. (Redrawn from [9].)

DIETARY FIBRE AND LIPID METABOLISM IN HUMANS 73

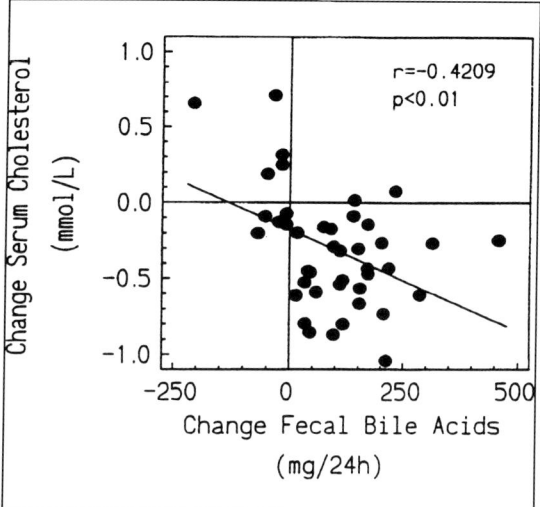

Figure 5. Relation between the difference in plasma total cholesterol and the difference in daily faecal bile acid excretion between the soluble and insoluble fibre diets. Values represent difference in measurements in 42 subjects. (Redrawn from [9]).

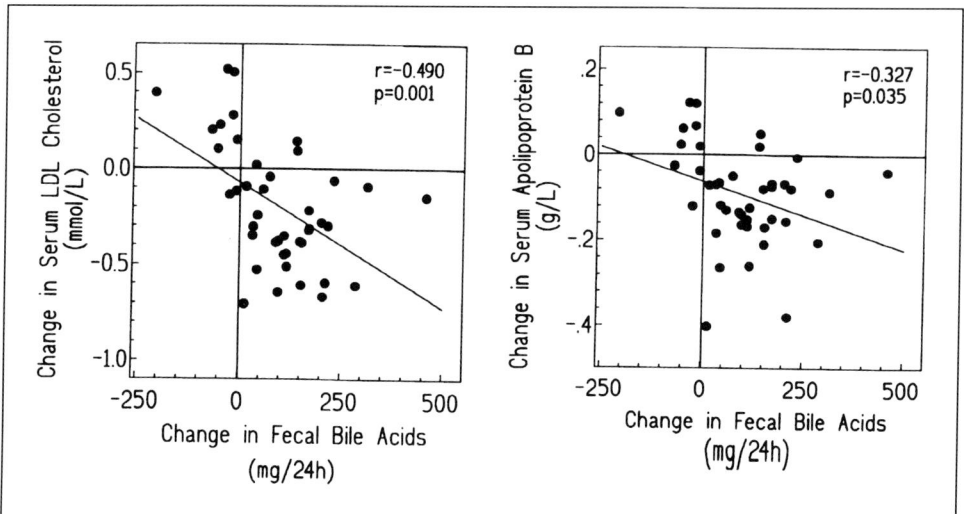

Figure 6. Relation between the difference in plasma LDL cholesterol (left) or B apolipoprotein (right) and the difference in daily faecal bile acid excretion between the soluble and insoluble fibre diets. Values represent difference in measurements in 42 subjects.

sources of either soluble or insoluble fibre in random order, with each diet lasting for four months [9]. The soluble fibre diet significantly reduced serum cholesterol *(Figure 3)* and increased faecal bile acid excretion *(Figure 4)*. In this study, there was a significant relationship between the change in faecal bile acid excretion and the change in total and LDL serum cholesterol *(Figures 5 and 6)*. In addition, there was a relationship between the change in faecal bile acid excretion and the change in apolipoprotein B *(Figure 6)*. These results support the hypothesis that increased faecal bile acid loss promoted by soluble fibre lowers serum cholesterol by increasing bile acid synthesis from hepatic cholesterol, thus reducing the intracellular pool of cholesterol, upregulating LDL receptors, and increasing hepatic uptake of plasma LDL particles.

Different fibers may have different effects on bile acid excretion which are not always related in consistent ways to cholesterol absorption, cholesterol synthesis and serum cholesterol. Miettinen and Tarpila [10] showed that guar gum and psyllium were associated with reduced serum cholesterol, increased faecal bile acid output, increased cholesterol synthesis and no change in cholesterol absorption *(Figure 7)*. The reduction in serum cholesterol in by these fibers was suggested to be due to intrahepatic cholesterol depletion, upregulation of hepatic LDL receptors and thus an increased removal of cholesterol from blood. By contrast, a high wheat fiber diet had no effect on serum cholesterol, but was associated with reduced faecal bile acid excretion, reduced cholesterol absorption and increased cholesterol synthesis. Anderson and others found that, in hypercholesterolaemic men, oat bran had the same cholesterol lowering effect as beans, but that these fibre sources had opposite effects on faecal bile acid excretion [11]. Studies such as these suggest that dietary fibre influences serum cholesterol by other mechanisms besides increases in faecal bile acid excretion. Indeed in our long-term metabolic studies *(Figures 3-6)* changes in faecal bile acid excretion accounted for only about 20 % of the variability in the change in serum cholesterol.

Altered lipid absorption

Dietary fibre has been suggested to reduce triglyceride and cholesterol absorption by binding bile acids and thus reducing micelle formation or by physically impairing digestion and absorption due to increased viscosity of the small intestinal contents [12-14]. In addition, dietary fibre may be associated with lipase inhibitors or other factors which may reduce fat absorption [15, 16]. Thus, a reduced amount or rate of lipid absorption could contribute to the cholesterol lowering effect of fibre. However, there is no clear relationship between the effect of different fibers on postprandial lipaemia and their cholesterol lowering effects. Both wheat bran, which does not reduce fasting serum cholesterol, and oat bran, which does lower serum cholesterol, have been shown to reduce the postprandial plasma triglyceride and cholesterol responses when added to fatty test meals [17]. On the other hand, a mixture of guar and oat bran has been reported to increase postprandial triglycerides, more so in women than men [18]. In addition, studies in experimental animals suggest that there is a long-term adaptation to the acute interference with fat absorption involving pancreatic hypertrophy and increased lipase and bile acid excretion [19]. These changes would tend to reduce fat malabsorption which might otherwise occur with dietary fibre. Most studies in humans have shown that, in the absence of pancreatic insufficiency, increased intake of dietary fibre causes a statistically significant but small increase in faecal fat excretion [20].

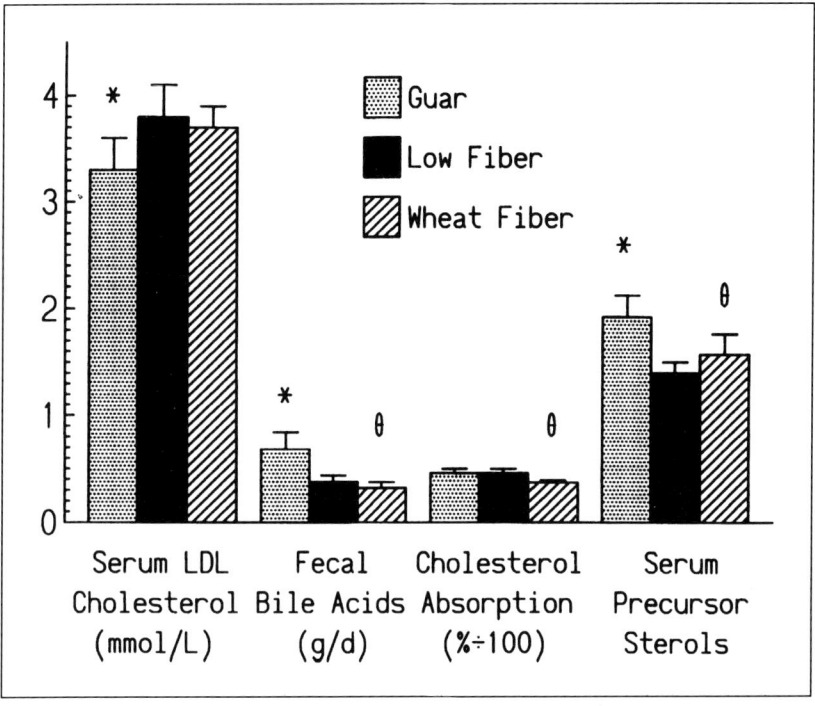

Figure 7. Effect of fibre serum LDL cholesterol concentrations, faecal bile acid excretion, cholesterol absorption and the concentration of cholesterol precursors in serum.
* : significant difference between guar and low fibre ; θ : significant difference between wheat fibre and low fibre. (Drawn from data presented in [10].)

We studied the long-term effect of soluble *versus* insoluble fibre on fat absorption and metabolism. After 14 to 16 weeks on each diet, subjects were given a fibre-free liquid test meal consisting of 0.5 g/kg body weight corn oil, 0.5g/kg glucose and 0.5g/kg protein from skimmed milk powder, plus 50,000IU retinyl palmitate as a marker of triglyceride-rich lipoprotein metabolism. The postprandial area under the chylomicron triglyceride curve was 22 ± 9 % ($p < 0.02$) greater after soluble *versus* insoluble fibre. When the subjects were separated according to their apolipoprotein E genotype, the increase in chylomicron triglyceride was seen in subjects with E3/E3 genotype, and not in those with E3/E4 or E4/E4. We used the kinetic model of Anh Le (personal communication) for kinetic analysis of the retinyl palmitate responses *(Figure 8)*. Since the soluble fibre diet was associated with increased faecal bile acid excretion, this suggested that there might be an expanded bile acid pool, leading to an increased rate of fat absorption and chylomicron formation (parameters P(31), P(1), L(3,2) and P(2)). There was some evidence for this, in that in the subjects with E3/E3 genotype, in whom there was a significant increase in postprandial chylomicron triglycerides, parameters P(1) and P(2) were significantly higher on soluble than insoluble fibre. However, when data for all the subjects was combined, there was no relationship between the change in faecal bile acid output and the change in any of the absorption parameters from the kinetic model. This suggests that other factors such as increased lipase secretion may have

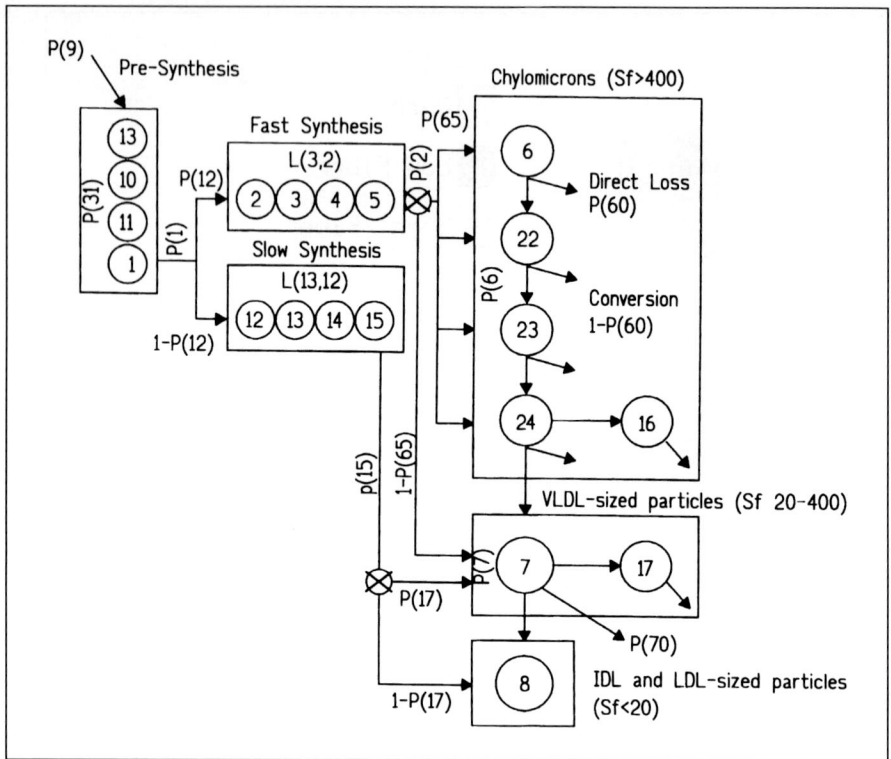

Figure 8. Kinetic model for postprandial triglyceride-rich lipoprotein metabolism.

also been associated with the changes in postprandial triglyceridaemia we observed. As discussed above, an increase in faecal bile acid excretion is hypothesized to reduce serum cholesterol by increasing the rate of hepatic uptake of LDL particles. It was of interest that the kinetic model provided evidence for this because the change in faecal bile acid excretion on soluble fibre was significantly related to the rate of transfer from pool 7 to pool 8, *i.e.* L(8,7), which represents the rate of conversion of chylomicron remnants to LDL particles, which presumably would also be related to the rate of removal of LDL by the liver.

Reduced insulin-stimulated cholesterol synthesis

Viscous dietary fibres which reduce serum cholesterol, such as guar and psyllium, also reduce blood glucose and insulin responses after meals, an effect which is not seen with non-viscous fibres such as wheat bran which do not reduce serum cholesterol [21, 22]. Since insulin is involved in the regulation of cholesterol synthesis in the liver [23], reduced postprandial insulin has been suggested as a possible way in which soluble fibre reduces cholesterol. Viscous fibre has been hypothesized to reduce postprandial insulin by slowing the rate of absorption of carbohydrate [24]. Increased meal frequency was used as a model to study the effects of slowing absorption without alteration in the nature of the food consumed and thus presumably no alteration in the amount of fat absorbed or the degree of colonic fermentation [25]. Nibbling was shown to result in about a 30 % reduction in mean day-long serum insulin concentration [26], and as much as a 15 % reduction in fasting serum cholesterol [27, 28]. Recently, it has been shown that the rate of cholesterol synthesis was reduced by nibbling [29]. Thus, there is good evidence that reducing mean serum insulin levels will reduce cholesterol synthesis and serum cholesterol levels.

What is the evidence that dietary fibre reduces serum insulin concentrations? When viscous fibre is added to single test meals, reductions in blood glucose and insulin responses are seen [30]. In addition, early studies showed that insulin requirements could be reduced in patients with diabetes on long-term guar [31], and more recently we have shown that a low-glycaemic index diet reduces urinary C-peptide excretion in normal [32] and diabetic [33] subjects. Nevertheless, there are few studies which have looked at the long-term effects of fibre on day-long serum insulin levels. There is some evidence that guar gum has little or no effect on mean serum insulin, although in this study there was also no effect of guar on blood glucose responses. Nevertheless, there was a marked reduction in mean serum GIP concentrations, and, paradoxically, a marked increase in serum C-peptide on guar, suggesting that guar increases insulin secretion and increases hepatic insulin extraction [34]. More recently, the same group has demonstrated in type 2 diabetic subjects on long-term guar therapy, that serum insulin responses were reduced initially, but that with prolonged treatment for 48 weeks, insulin and C-peptide responses increased, suggesting that a long-term adaptation to guar occurred resulting in increased insulin secretion [35]. Since guar reduced mean blood glucose levels, it is possible that the increase in insulin secretion represents the reduced effects of glucose toxicity on the pancreatic β-cell [36].

In our studies with mixed soluble and insoluble fibre diets, it was unlikely that reduced insulin played any role in the cholesterol-lowering effect we observed. There was only a small difference between the calculated glycaemic index values of the soluble and insoluble fibre diets, which was reflected in a small reduction in the area under the blood glucose response curve on soluble fibre, and no significant reduction of serum insulin concentrations throughout the day.

Colonic short chain fatty acids

Some purified forms of fibre which lower serum cholesterol, such as oat bran, guar and pectin, are readily fermented in the colon with the production of the short chain fatty acids acetate, propionate and butyrate. Butyrate is present in portal blood in only trace amounts because it is believed to be taken up by the colonic mucosa and used as a major fuel. However, acetate and propionate are readily absorbed and it has been suggested that acetate and propionate may lower serum cholesterol by inhibiting hepatic cholesterol synthesis. Acetate has been shown to inhibit cholesterol synthesis from lactate, and the reduction in serum cholesterol by oat bran is accompanied by an increase in serum acetate. Nevertheless, it is not clear that acetate actually reduces cholesterol synthesis because it is the primary substrate for cholesterol synthesis and is readily incorporated into cholesterol in isolated hepatocytes. In addition, acetate has no effect on the rate of incorporation of deuterium or tritium into cholesterol, which are considered by most to be the most accurate method of determining overall cholesterol synthesis.

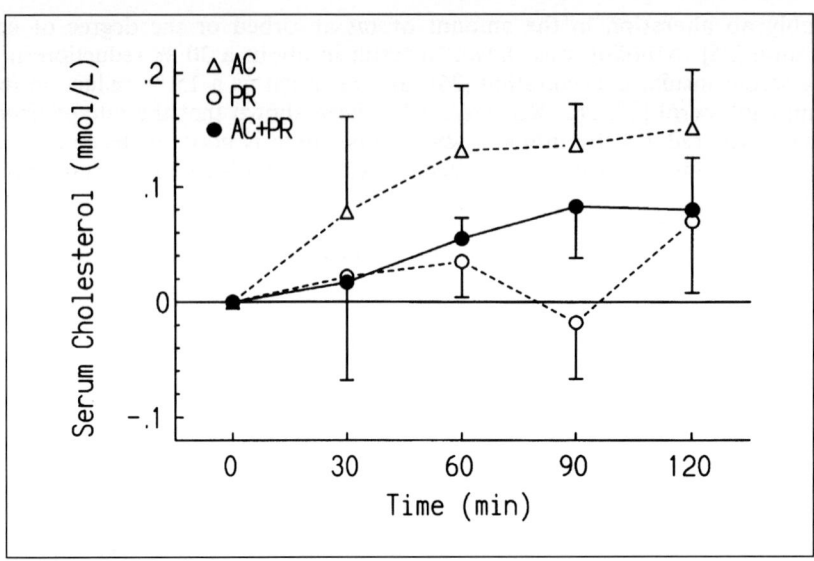

Figure 9. Effect of rectal infusion of 180 mmoles acetate (AC), 180 mmoles proprionate (PR) or 180 mmoles acetate plus 60 mmoles proprionate (AC + PR) on total serum cholesterol in healthy subjects. Values are mean ± SEM increments relative to the saline control. (Redrawn from [38].)

Propionate also has been shown to inhibit cholesterol synthesis from acetate in isolated hepatic cells *in vitro*. There is some controversy as to whether the concentration of propionate in portal blood is high enough to inhibit cholesterol synthesis and animal studies suggest that propionate reduces serum cholesterol by redistributing cholesterol from blood to liver or adipose tissue. Two human studies have shown that propionate had no significant effect on serum cholesterol. However, a recent study by Stephen *et al.* [37] using a larger dose of propionate did show an effect. It was hypothesized that the effect of propionate might be due to propionate binding with carnitine and thus reducing its availability for transporting fatty acids across the mitochondrial membrane. However, the reduction in serum cholesterol seen on propionate was not associated with any change in serum or urine carnitine levels [37].

Studies from our laboratory suggest that the effect of short chain fatty acids on lipid metabolism may depend upon the relative amounts of acetate and propionate produced. Rectal infusion of 180 mmoles acetate has been shown to increase serum cholesterol within 1 hour, an effect which was partly blocked by adding 60 mmoles propionate [38] *(Figure 9)*. In addition, the incorporation of rectally infused ^{13}C-acetate into serum cholesterol and triglycerides was blocked by adding propionate [39]. The results of these somewhat unphysiologic experiments were confirmed by a study in which healthy subjects were given 25 g lactulose daily for 2 weeks. Lactulose, an unabsorbed sugar which has been shown to produce a large proportion of acetate when fermented *in vitro*, significantly increased fasting total and LDL cholesterol and apolipoprotein B concentrations when compared to an identical metabolically controlled low fat diet [40]. There was also some support for a possible serum cholesterol raising effect of acetate in our studies with soluble and insoluble fibre. After the subjects had been on the diets for 14 weeks, serum acetate and plasma LDL cholesterol concentrations were measured over an 8 hour period during the day on the actual study diets. Plasma LDL cholesterol was significantly lower through the day on soluble than insoluble fibre. Fasting serum acetate was significantly higher on the soluble than insoluble fibre diet, but postprandial serum acetate concentrations tended to be lower on the soluble than the insoluble fibre diet and there was no difference in the overall mean daily concentration. Nevertheless, there was a significant positive correlation between the change in mean daily serum acetate on the soluble *versus* insoluble fibre diet and the change mean daily serum LDL cholesterol.

Conclusions

There is evidence that dietary fibre may influence serum cholesterol by at least four mechanisms : increased faecal bile acid excretion, altered fat absorption, reduced insulin-stimulated cholesterol synthesis, and the effects of colonic short chain fatty acids. However, different types of fibre may reduce serum cholesterol by different mechanisms. In addition, these mechanisms are not mutually exclusive, and may even act in opposite directions in any particular case.

Summary

At least four mechanisms have been proposed to explain the cholesterol-lowering effect of soluble fiber : (1) increased faecal bile acid excretion ; (2) altered lipid absorption ; (3) reduced insulin stimulus to cholesterol synthesis ; and (4) effects of colonic short chain fatty acids. The serum cholesterol concentration reflects a balance between the rate of cholesterol input into the blood (absorption from the gut, and synthesis in the liver) and the rate of cholesterol removal from the blood (uptake by peripheral tissues ; uptake by liver for secretion into bile or conversion to bile acids). Recent studies have established that soluble fibre increases faecal bile acid output which may actually be associated with increased hepatic cholesterol synthesis. The fall in serum cholesterol appears to be due to an increase in bile acid synthesis associated with increased faecal bile acid loss. Fibre or associated food factors (*e.g.* enzyme inhibitors) may reduce lipid absorption acutely resulting in reduced postprandial triglyceride and cholesterol responses. However, long-term adaptation may occur with increased bile acid and digestive enzyme secretion and enhanced postprandial chylomicron triglyceride responses. Reducing mean plasma insulin by increased meal frequency is associated with reduced serum cholesterol and reduced hepatic cholesterol synthesis. However, changes in mean plasma insulin on soluble fibre, if any, are small. Nevertheless, soluble fibre may affect other hormones which influence lipid metabolism directly or indirectly, including reduced plasma GIP, increased insulin secretion and increased hepatic insulin clearance. Fermentation of dietary fibre in the colon produces the short chain fatty acids acetate and propionate which have been suggested to reduce cholesterol synthesis. However, there is evidence that colonic acetate raises serum cholesterol, but that propionate blocks this effect, possibly by inhibiting the incorporation of acetate into serum cholesterol. Thus, the effect of colonic fermentation on serum cholesterol may depend upon the relative amounts of acetate and propionate produced.

Supported by : the Natural Sciences and Engineering Research Council of Canada, the Heart, Lung, and Blood Institute, National Institutes of Health (RO 1 HL 39689), Kellogg Canada Inc, and Loblaw Companies Limited.

References

1. Jenkins DJA, Spadafora PJ, Jenkins AL, Rainey-Macdonald CG. Fiber in the treatment of hyperlipidemia. In : Spiller GA, ed. *CRC Handbook of dietary fiber in human nutrition.* 2nd ed. Boca Raton, Florida : CRC Press, Inc, 1993 : 419-38.
2. Trowell HC. Ischemic heart disease and dietary fiber. *Am J Clin Nutr* 1972 ; 25 : 926-32
3. Kritchevsky D, Story JA. Binding of bile salts *in vitro* by nonnutritive fiber. *J Nutr* 1974 ; 104 : 458-62.
4. Story JA, Kritchevsky D. Comparison of the binding of various bile acids and bile salts by several types of fiber. *J Nutr* 1976 ; 106 : 1292-4.
5. Story JA, Furumoto. Dietary fiber and bile acid metabolism. In : Kritchevsly D, Bonfield C, Anderson JW eds. *Dietary fiber : chemistry, physiology, and health effects.* New York : Plenum Press, 1990 : 365-74.
6. Story JA. Dietary fiber and lipid metabolism. *Proc Soc Exp Biol Med* 1985 ; 180 : 447-52.
7. Anderson JW, Deakins DA, Bridges SR. Soluble fiber : hypocholesterolemic effects and proposed mechanisms. In : Kritchevsky D, Bonfield C, Anderson JW, eds. *Dietary fiber : chemistry, physiology, and health effects.* New York : Plenum Press, 1990 : 339-63.
8. Everson GT, Daggy BP, McKinley C, Story JA. Effects of psyllium hydrophillic mucilloid on LDL-cholesterol and bile acid synthesis in hypercholesterolemic men. *J Lipid Res* 1992 ; 33 : 1183-92.
9. Jenkins DJA, Wolever TMS, Rao AV, Hegele RA, Mitchell S, Ransom T, Boctor D, Spadafora PJ, Mehling C, Katzman Relle L, Connelly PW, Story JA, Furumoto EJ, Corey P, Würsch P. Effect on serum lipids of very high fiber intakes in diets low in saturated fat and cholesterol. *N Engl J Med* 1993 ; 329 : 21-6.
10. Miettinen TA, Tarpila S. Serum lipids and cholesterol metabolism during guar gum, plantago ovata and high fibre treatments. *Clin Chim Acta* 1989 ; 183 : 253-62.
11. Anderson JW, Story L, Sieling B, Chen WJ, Petro MS, Story J. Hypocholesterolemic effects of oat-bran and bean intake for hypercholesterolemic men. *Am J Clin Nutr* 1984 ; 40 : 1146-55.
12. Vahouny GV, Satchithanandam S, Chen I, Tepper SA, Kritchevsky D, Lightfoot FG, Cassidy MM. Dietary fiber and intestinal adaptation : effects on lipid absorption and lymphatic transport in the rat. *Am J Clin Nutr* 1988 ; 47 : 201-6.
13. Borel P, Lairon D, Senft M, Chautan M, Lafont H. Wheat bran and wheat germ : effect on digestion and intestinal absorption of dietary lipids in the rat. *Am J Clin Nutr* 1989 ; 49 : 1192-202.
14. Ebihara K, Schneeman BO. Interaction of bile acids, phospholipids, cholesterol and triglyceride with dietary fibers in the small intestine of rats. *J Nutr* 1989 ; 119 : 1100-6.
15. Lairon D, Lafont H, Vigne JL, Nalbone G, Léonardi J, Houton JC. Effects of dietary fibers and cholestyramine on the activity of pancreatic lipase *in vitro*. *Am J Clin Nutr* 1985 ; 42 : 629-38.
16. Borel P, Lairon D, Termine E, Grataroli R, Lafont H. Isolation and properties of lipolysis inhibitory proteins from wheat germ and wheat bran. *Plant Foods Hum Nutr* 1989 ; 39 : 339-48.
17. Cara L, Dubois C, Borel P, Armand M, Senft M, Portugal H, Pauli AM, Bernard PM, Lairon D. Effects of oat bran, rice bran, wheat fiber, and wheat germ on postprandial lipemia in healthy adults. *Am J Clin Nutr* 1992 ; 55 : 81-8.
18. Redard CL, Davis PA, Schneeman BO. Dietary fiber and gender : effect on postprandial lipemia. *Am J Clin Nutr* 1990 ; 52 : 837-45.
19. Ikegami S, Tsuchihashi F, Harada H, Tsuchihashi N, Nishide E, Innami S. Effect of viscous indigestible polysaccharides on pancreatic-biliary secretion and digestive organs in rats. *J Nutr* 1990 ; 120 : 353-60.
20. Cummings JH. The effect of dietary fiber on fecal weight and composition. In : Spiller GA, ed. *CRC handbook of dietary fiber in human nutrition.* 2nd ed. Boca Raton, Florida : CRC Press, Inc, 1993 : 263-349.
21. Jenkins DJA, Wolever TMS, Leeds AR, Gassull MA, Dilawari JB, Goff DV, Metz GL,

Alberti KGMM. Dietary fibres, fibre analogues and glucose tolerance : importance of viscosity. *Br Med J* 1978 ; 1 : 1392-4.
22. Pastors JG, Blaisdell PW, Balm TK, Asplin CM, Pohl SL. Psyllium fiber reduces rise in postprandial glucose and insulin concentrations in patients with non-insulin-dependent diabetes. *Am J Clin Nutr* 1991 ; 53 : 1431-5.
23. Rodwell VW, Nordstrom JL, Mitschelen JJ. Regulation of HMG-CoA reductase. *Adv Lipid Res* 1976 ; 14 : 1-76.
24. Blackburn NA, Redfern JS, JarJis M, Holgate AM, Manning I, Scarpello JHB, Johnson IT, Read NW. The mechanism of action of guar gum in improving glucose tolerance in man. *Clin Sci* 1984 ; 66 : 329-36.
25. Brighenti F, Ciappellano S, Vuksan V, Rao AV, Wolever TMS, Jenkins A, Jenkins DJA, Testolin. Is colonic fermentation minimized by increasing meal frequency ? *Eur J Clin Nutr* 1991 ; 45 : 221-31.
26. Wolever TMS. Metabolic effects of continuous feeding. *Metabolism* 1990 ; 39 : 947-51.
27. Jenkins DJA, Wolever TMS, Vuksan V, Brighenti F, Cunnane SC, Rao AV, Jenkins A, Buckley G, Patten R, Singer W, Corey P, Josse RG. « Nibbling versus gorging » : metabolic advantages of increased meal frequency. *N Engl J Med* 1989 ; 321 : 929-34.
28. Arnold LM, Ball MJ, Duncan AW, Mann J. Effect of isoenergetic intake of three or nine meals on plasma lipoproteins and glucose metabolism. *Am J Clin Nutr* 1993 ; 57 : 446-51.
29. Jones PJH, Leitch CA, Pederson RA. Meal-frequency effects on plasma hormone concentrations and cholesterol synthesis in humans. *Am J Clin Nutr* 1993 ; 57 : 868-74.
30. Wolever TMS, Jenkins DJA. Effect of dietary fiber and foods on carbohydrate metabolism. In : Spiller GA, ed. *CRC handbook of dietary fiber in human nutrition.* 2nd ed. Boca Raton, Florida : CRC Press, Inc, 1993 : 111-52.
31. Jenkins DJA, Wolever TMS, Taylor RH, Reynolds D, Nineham R, Hockaday TDR. Diabetic glucose control, lipids, and trace elements on long term guar. *Br Med J* 1980 ; 1 : 1353-4.
32. Jenkins DJA, Wolever TMS, Collier GR, Ocana A, Rao AV, Buckley G, Lam KY, Meyer A, Thompson LU. The metabolic effects of a low glycemic index diet. *Am J Clin Nutr* 1987 ; 46 : 968-75.
33. Wolever TMS, Jenkins DJA, Vuksan V, Jenkins AL, Buckley GC, Wong GS, Josse RG. Beneficial effect of a low-glycaemic index diet in type 2 diabetes. *Diab Med* 1992 ; 9 : 451-8.
34. Groop PH, Groop L, Totterman KJ, Fyhrquist F. Relationship between changes in GIP concentrations and changes in insulin and c-peptide concentrations after guar gum therapy. *Scand J Clin Lab Invest* 1986 ; 46 : 505-10.
35. Groop PH, Aro A, Stenman S, Groop L. Long-term effects of guar gum in subjects with non-insulin-dependent diabetes mellitus. *Am J Clin Nutr* 1993 ; 58 : 513-8.
36. Rossetti L, Giaccari A, DeFronzo RA. Glucose toxicity. *Diabetes Care* 1990 ; 13 : 610-30.
37. Stephen A. Propionate — sources and effect on lipid metabolism. In : Binder HJ, Cummings JH, Soergel KH, eds. *Short chain fatty acids / Falk Symposium 73* 1994 : 260-71.
38. Wolever TMS, Spadafora P, Eshuis H. Interaction between colonic acetate and propionate in man. *Am J Clin Nutr* 1991 ; 53 : 681-7.
39. Wolever TMS, Spadafora PJ, Cunnane SC, Pencharz PB. Unpublished.
40. Jenkins DJA, Wolever TMS, Jenkins A, Brighenti F, Vuksan V, Rao AV, Cunnane SC, Ocana A, Corey P, Versina C, Connelly P, Buckley G, Patten R. Specific types of colonic fermentation may raise low-density-lipoprotein-cholesterol concentrations. *Am J Clin Nutr* 1991 ; 54 : 141-7.

8

Fibre effect on nutrient metabolism in splanchnic and peripheral tissues

B. DARCY-VRILLON, P.H. DUEE

*Unité d'Écologie et de Physiologie du Système Digestif,
Institut National de la Recherche Agronomique,
Jouy-en-Josas, France.*

Dietary fibre (DF) in the human diet is essentially present as nonstarch polysaccharides, together with a fraction of starch, namely resistant starch, and some oligosaccharides. According to Cummings and Englyst [1], « DF is a valuable nutritional concept embodying the resistance to digestion in the small intestine of plant cell wall material, which decreases the rate of carbohydrate and lipid absorption, and exerts a beneficial effect on large intestinal function by acting as a substrate for fermentation ». This definition provides the basis for considering the mechanisms by which DF can affect nutrient metabolism at the cellular level.

The alteration of nutrient absorption and hormonal response has been observed consistently for soluble, viscous fibres. Several studies have shown the decrease of blood glucose and insulin responses to test-meals enriched with guar gum and pectin [2-4]. This effect provides the basis for the commonly used glycemic index, expressing the post-prandial glycemic area of a test-product as a percentage of the corresponding area of glucose or white-bread [5, 6]. Finally, prolonged post-prandial reductions in nutrient fluxes and insulin secretion may affect cellular and overall carbohydrate or lipid metabolism [7].

Fermentation in the large intestine is the second mechanism by which fibre can affect nutrient metabolism. It has been hypothetized that some of the reported effects of soluble DF, which cannot be explained by the slowing down of nutrient absorption after a meal, could be mediated by the short chain fatty acids (SCFA) produced by bacterial colonic fermentation. In the present review, we will discuss how and where these SCFA (acetate, propionate and butyrate) are metabolized, and how this can affect carbohydrate and lipid metabolism.

Table I. SCFA concentrations (µmol/L ± SEM) in pig and human blood.

	Pig after 12 hr fasting (Rérat et al., 1987)	
	Portal	Arterial
Acetate	548 ± 23	178 ± 10
Propionate	281 ± 11	14 ± 1
Butyrate	71 ± 2	9 ± 1

	Human at autopsy (Cummings et al., 1987)		
	Portal	Hepatic	Arterial
Acetate	258 ± 40	115 ± 28	70 ± 19
Propionate	88 ± 28	21 ± 10	5 ± 2
Butyrate	29 ± 8	12 ± 4	4 ± 2

Site of SCFA metabolism

Circulating SCFA concentrations measured in various blood vessels of pigs or humans *(Table I)* point out to the splanchnic area as the main site of SCFA utilization. In peripheral blood, there are very low levels of propionate and butyrate, whereas higher acetate concentrations can be detected. Thus, this indicates that propionate and butyrate are almost totally cleared by the splanchnic area, whereas acetate partly escapes. The low butyrate concentrations in the portal blood suggest that butyrate is essentially metabolized in the intestine ; propionate would be essentially cleared by the liver.

Metabolic fate of SCFA in the digestive epithelium

SCFA produced in the colon first get transported across the large intestinal epithelium. Indeed SCFA transport, which has been shown to be rapid and not saturable, should therefore not be limiting for their subsequent metabolism. Two possible mechanisms have been hypothetized transport under ionic *vs* non ionic form — and are still actively investigated [8, 9].

Metabolic fate of butyrate in colonocytes

Even if the capacities to utilize butyrate differ somewhat between species, the ratio between oxidation and ketogenesis is more or less constant : CO_2 production accounts for around 40 % of butyrate metabolism and total ketone body (TKB) production for the remaining 60 % *(Figure 1)*. In all species, aceto-acetate represents 70 % to 80 % of the ketone bodies generated. Some regional differences can be observed in the human colon *(Figure 1)* : there is more CO_2 and less TKB produced in the distal part of the colon.

The metabolic pathways involved in butyrate utilization in colonocytes are shown in *Figure 2*. Butyrate gets first activated in the mitochondria by a butyryl-CoA-synthetase which specificity towards butyrate is not clearly established. Butyryl-CoA

FIBRE EFFECT ON NUTRIENT METABOLISM IN SPLANCHNIC AND PERIPHERAL TISSUES   85

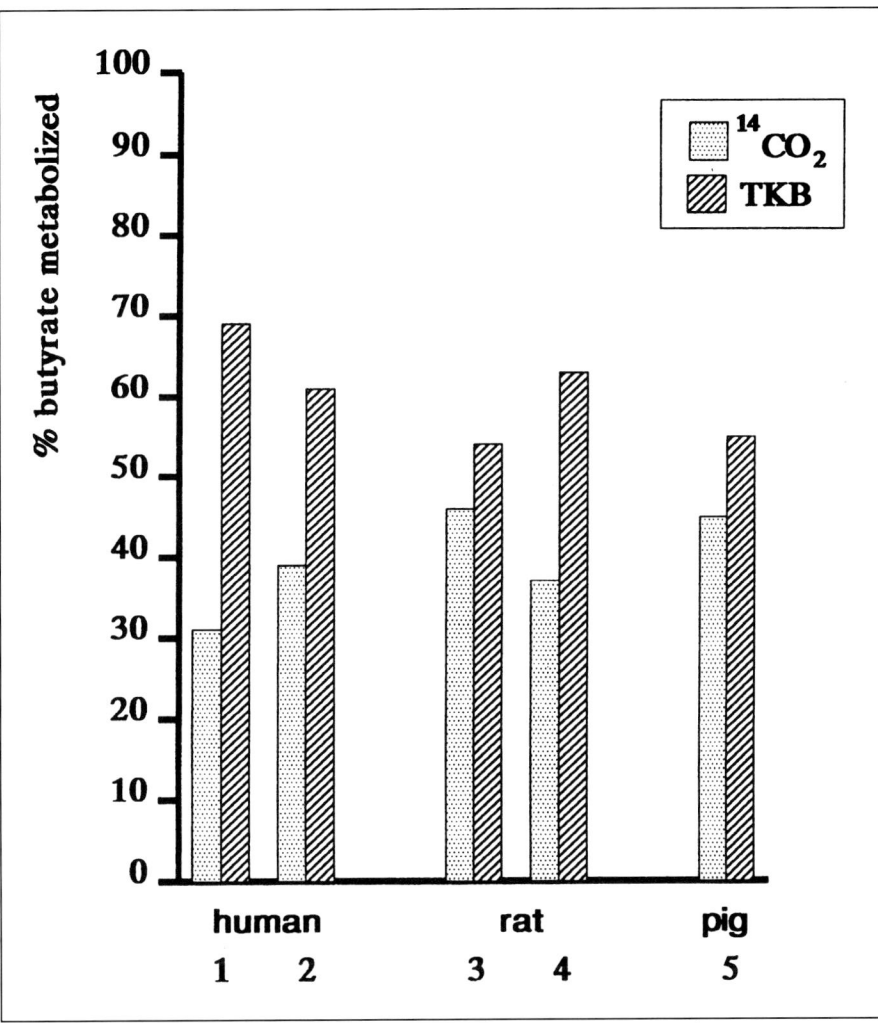

Figure 1. Metabolic fate of butyrate in isolated epithelial colonic cells. 1 : human ascending colon [13] ; 2 : human descending colon [13] ; 3 : rat [14] ; 4 : rat [17] ; 5 : pig proximal colon [20]. TKB = Total ketone bodies.

follows the β-oxidation pathways generating acetoacetyl-CoA. The latter can be cleaved by the acetyl-CoA acetyl transferase or thiolase, to generate acetyl-CoA which can enter the TCA cycle or condense with aceto-acetyl-CoA to enter the hydroxymethyl-glutaryl-CoA (HMgCoA) cycle. The HMgCoA synthase pathway would be the major route for ketogenesis in the colon [10, 11], (Darcy-Vrillon et al., unpublished data). Accordingly, the other pathways which predominate in the rumen of ruminants (aceto-acetyl deacylase ; 3-ketoacid CoA transferase) would be

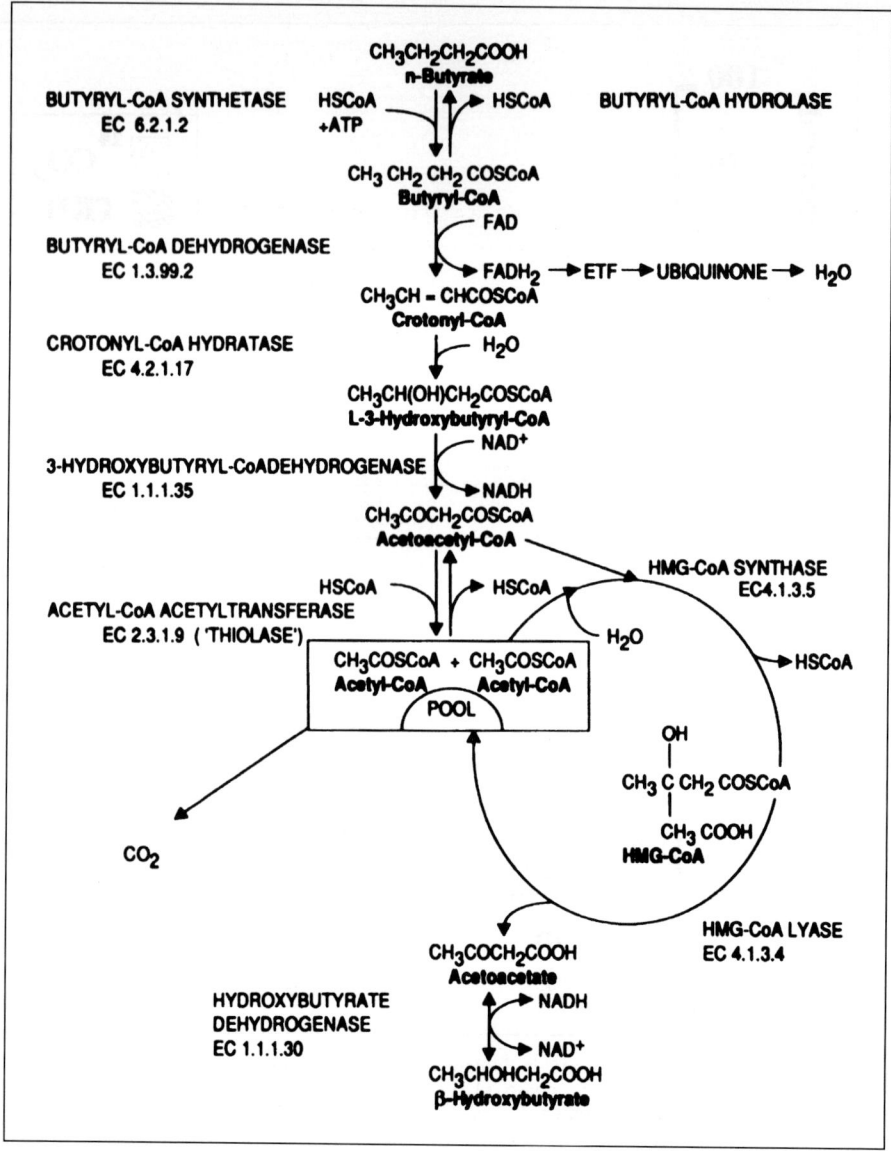

Figure 2. Pathways of n-butyrate oxidation to acetyl-CoA, acetoacetate and β-hydroxybutyrate. (Adapted from [11].)
HMg-CoA = 3-hydroxy-3-methyl-glutaryl-CoA

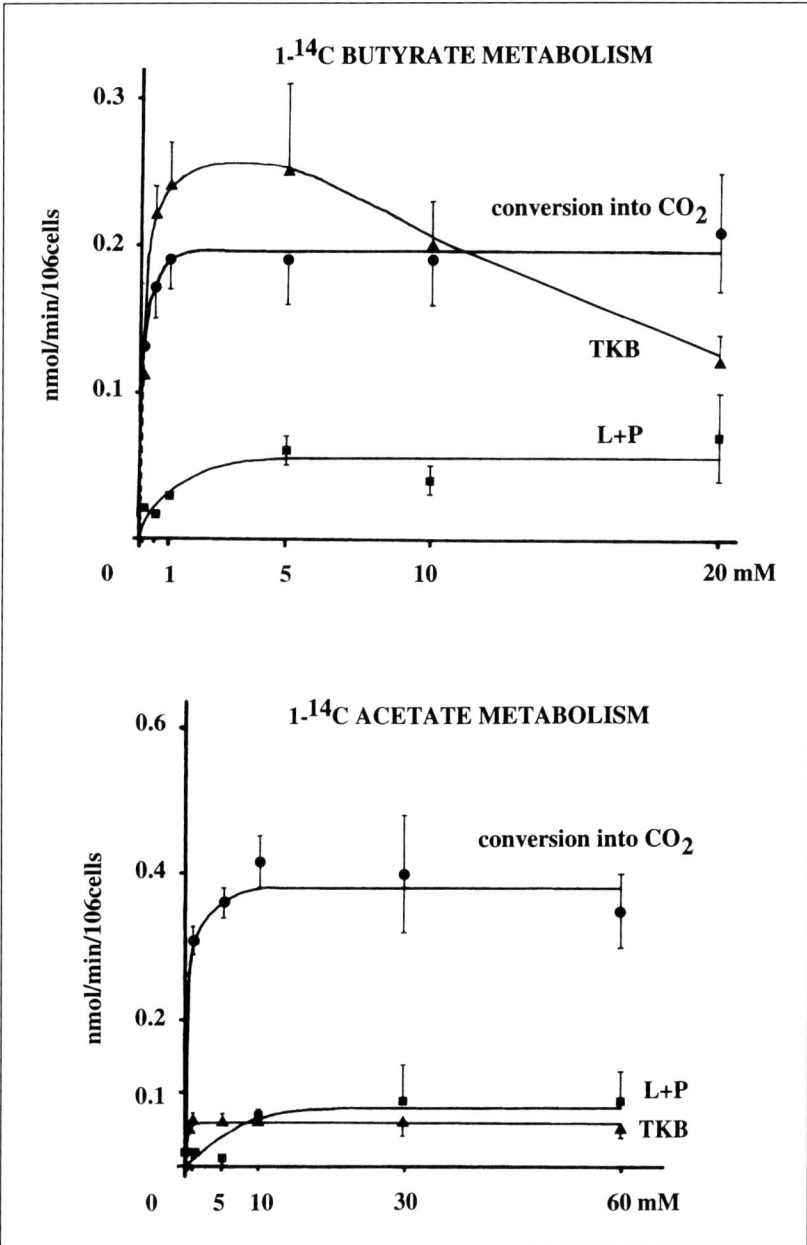

Figure 3. Concentration-dependence of butyrate and acetate metabolism in isolated colonic cells from the pig. Results are means ± SEM (n = 4) of butyrate or acetate conversion into $^{14}CO_2$, total ketone bodies (TKB), and lactate + pyruvate (L + P). Cell viability was not modified by adding increasing concentrations of butyrate or acetate.

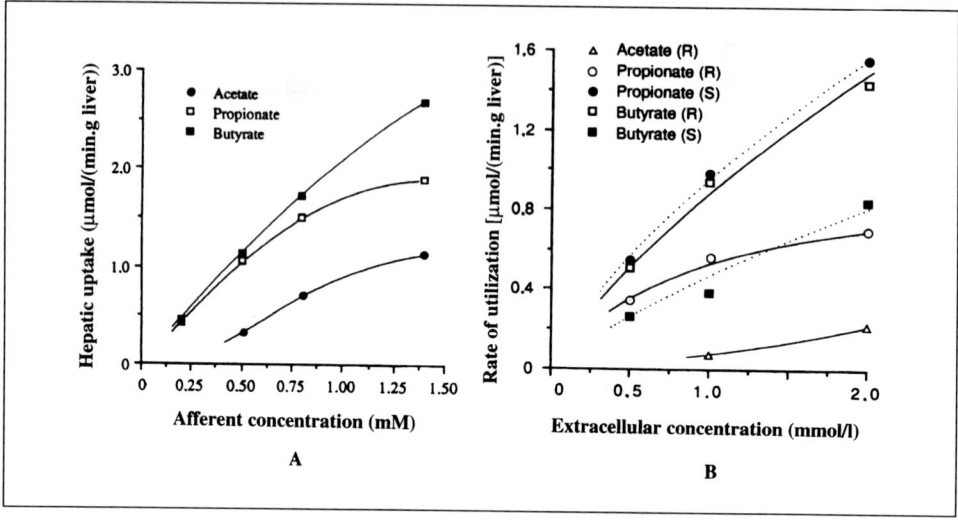

Figure 5. Concentration-dependence of short-chain fatty acid uptake by the post-absorptive liver. A : *in vivo* (from [26]). Concentrations of SCFA in the afferent plasma were modified by infusion of SCFA sodium salts *via* a mesenteric vein. B : *in vitro* (from [31]). Rates of propionate and butyrate utilization were measured in rat (R) or sheep (S) hepatocytes.

Hepatic balances of SCFA and impact on other nutrients

In rats adapted to a high fibre *vs* a fibre-free diet, and taken in the fed state [23], intestinal absorption of SCFA is greatly enhanced. Hepatic balances indicate that acetate reaching the liver is partly taken up, while propionate and butyrate are totally taken up. These changes are also accompanied by profound changes in glucose metabolism : when switching from a situation of high glucose absorption to a situation where no glucose is absorbed from the intestine, the hepatic balance also switches from glucose uptake to glucose release. Similar findings have been reported when digestible starch was replaced by resistant starch in the diet [24]. In the latter experiment, the increased production and metabolism of SCFA in the splanchnic area were accompanied by changes in glucose and lipid metabolism. Hepatic lipogenesis was found to be severely reduced during the fed period in rats receiving the resistant starch diet [25].

SCFA activation in the liver

Propionate and butyrate are almost exclusively activated in the mitochondrial matrix. In the rat, there is a propionyl CoA synthetase (Km ~ 0.2 mM) but no specific butyryl-CoA synthetase, butyrate being probably activated by a medium chain acyl-CoA synthetase [26]. The site of acetate activation, mitochondria *vs* cytosolic, is still debated. Scholte and Groot [27] described an acetyl-CoA synthetase activity both in liver cytosol (Km ~ 0.1 mM) and in liver mitochondria (Km ~ 10 mM). However, they reported that more than 80 % of the activity was present in the cytosol. More recently, Crabtree *et al.* [28] measured the rates of acetyl-CoA synthesis and hydrolysis. Even with 1mM acetate, they found that synthesis was much higher in the mitochondria than in the cytosol. In the latter, the net balance

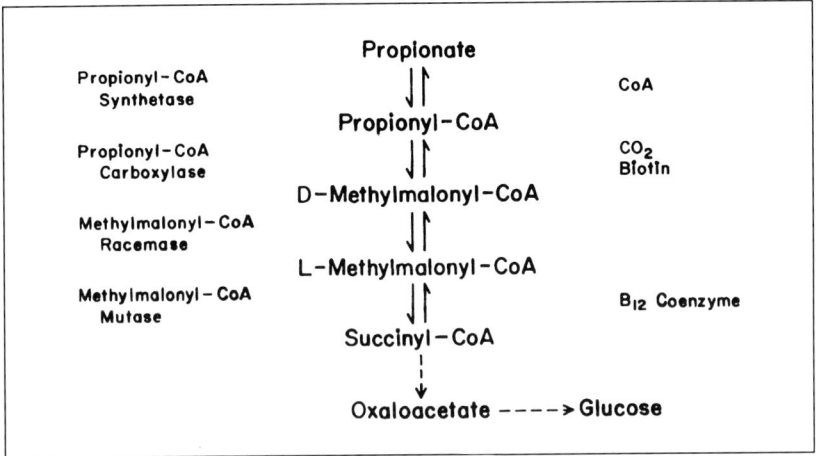

Figure 6. Major metabolic pathways for propionate in the liver. (From [26].)

was in favour of acetate production, hydrolysis of acetyl-CoA being much higher than synthesis.

Metabolic pathways of SCFA utilization

As observed in the colonic epithelium *(Figure 2)*, butyrate can generate acetyl-CoA or ketone bodies in the mitochondria. Acetate generates acetylCoA in the cytosol or in the mitochondria, thus directly or indirectly providing a precursor for lipogenesis. Propionate, entering the TCA cycle at the level of succinyl-CoA *(Figure 6)*, can be used as a neoglucogenic precursor. While this role is well established in ruminants, it is still debated for monogastric species. A net production of glucose from propionate has been evidenced in rat and rabbit hepatocytes [29, 30]. As compared to gluconeogenic precursors such as lactate or alanine, propionate by generating oxaloacetate bypasses the regulatory step of pyruvate carboxylase.

Metabolic interactions

Again interactions between SCFA must be considered. Acetate use is inhibitable by butyrate and propionate and by long chain fatty acids used for energy supply in the liver [26]. In rat and sheep hepatocytes [31], butyrate (1 or 2 mM) also reduces propionate (1 mM) consumption.

There are also important interactions between SCFA and other metabolic substrates. Besides the possible generation of glucose from propionate, SCFA also interfere with glucose metabolism by having an effect on neoglucogenesis from other substrates, *e.g.* lactate, or on glycolysis. In rat hepatocytes, gluconeogenesis from lactate could be enhanced by butyrate or acetate whereas it is inhibited by propionate [29, 32]. Conversely, lactate production from glucose was found to be inhibited by acetate or butyrate and stimulated by propionate [29].

Another important issue is how propionate can affect lipid metabolism. It has been proposed that propionate, by inhibiting *de novo* synthesis of cholesterol and fatty acids in the liver, could be a mediator of the hypocholesterolemic effect of some DF [33]. The exact mechanisms by which this inhibition could occur are still controverted [34, 35].

Effect of SCFA on peripheral and overall metabolism

Acetate is the only SCFA reaching peripheral tissues in significant amounts. It is used for oxidative or lipogenic purposes, mostly in muscles and adipose tissue [26]. Most of the information on the metabolic pathways of SCFA utilization and their effect on carbohydrate and lipid metabolism derives from animal studies. However, the effect of acetate and propionate on glucose and lipid metabolism has been investigated in several human studies [6, 36-38]. The most consistent effect reported is a reduction of free fatty acid blood level. Parameters of glucose metabolism, *i.e.* blood glucose, glucose turnover rate or hepatic glucose production, and blood cholesterol levels were unchanged in most studies. Several factors can be put forward to explain the discrepancies between *in vitro* and *in vivo* data : (1) the concentrations used in *in vitro* experiments can be higher than the physiological concentrations (ex : concentrations found in the portal vein) ; (2) the time-course of appearance in the liver is different for SCFA administered orally *vs* produced in the colon [39] ; (3) the metabolic fate of SCFA reaching the liver may differ according to the prevailing metabolic conditions : neoglucogenic *vs* lipogenic orientation...

In conclusion, while the digestive effects of DF are now well established, their metabolic effects still need to be documented. If the role of butyrate is easily evidenced in the colonic epithelium, further work is needed to clarify the effects of acetate and propionate on liver and peripheral tissues, especially in humans.

References

1. Cummings JH, Englyst HN. What is dietary fibre ? *Trends Food Sci Technol* 1991 ; 2 : 99-103.
2. Jenkins DJA, Goff DV, Leeds AR, Alberti KGMM, Wolever TMS, Gassull MA, Hockaday TDR. Unabsorbable carbohydrates and diabetes : decreased post-prandial hyperglycemia. *Lancet* 1976 ; 2 : 172-4.
3. Jenkins DJA, Wolever TMS, Leeds AR, Gassull MA, Haisman P, Dilawari J, Goff DV, Metz GL, Alberti KGMM. Dietary fibres, fibre analogues, and glucose tolerance : importance of viscosity. *Br Med J* 1978 ; 1 : 1392-4.
4. Torsdottir I, Alpsten M, Andersson H, Einarsson S. Dietary guar gum effects on postprandial blood glucose, insulin and hydroxyproline in humans. *J Nutr* 1989 ; 119 : 1925-31.
5. Wolever TMS, Jenkins DJA. The use of the glycemic index in predicting the blood glucose response to mixed meals. *Am J Clin Nutr* 1986 ; 43 : 167-72.
6. Wolever TMS, Jenkins DJA, Jankins AL, Josse RG. The glycemic index : methodology and clinical applications. *Am J Clin Nutr* 1991 ; 54 : 846-54.
7. Jenkins DJA, Wolever TMS, Collier GR, Ocana A, Venketeshwer RAO A, Buckley G, Lam Y, Mayer A, Thompson LU. Metabolic effects of a low-glycemic-index diet. *Am J Clin Nutr* 1987 ; 46 : 968-75.
8. Von Engelhardt W, Busche R, Gros G, Rechkemmer G. Absorption of short chain fatty acids : mechanisms and regional differences in the large intestine. In : Roche AF, ed.

Short chain fatty acids : metabolism and clinical importance. Report of the 10th Ross conference on medical research. Columbus, Ohio : Ross Laboratories, 1991 : 60-2.
9. Binder HJ, Sandle GI, Rajendran VM. Colonic fluid and electrolyte transport in health and disease. In : Phillips SF, Pemberton JH, Shorter RG, eds. *The large intestine. Physiology, pathophysiology and disease.* New York ; Raven Press, 1991 : 141-68.
10. Henning SJ, Hird FJR. Ketogenesis from butyrate and acetate by the caecum and the colon of rabbits. *Biochem J* 1972 ; 130 : 785-90.
11. Roediger WEW, Duncan A, Kapaniris O, Millard S. Sulphide impairment of substrate oxidation in rat colonocytes : a biochemical basis for ulcerative colitis ? *Clin Sci* 1993 ; 85 : 623-7.
12. Roediger WEW, Kapaniris O, Millard S. Lipogenesis from n-butyrate in colonocytes. Action of reducing agent and 5-aminosalicylic acid with relevance to ulcerative colitis. *Mol Cell Biochem* 1992 ; 118 : 113-8.
13. Roediger WEW. Role of anaerobic bacteria in the metabolic welfare of the colonic mucosa in man. *Gut* 1980 ; 21 : 793-8.
14. Roediger WEW. Utilization of nutrients by isolated epithelial cells of the rat colon. *Gastroenterology* 1982 ; 83 : 424-9.
15. Kight CE, Fleming SE. Nutrient oxidation by rat intestinal epithelial cells is concentration dependent. *J Nutr* 1993 ; 123 : 876-82.
16. Watford M, Lund P, Krebs HA. Isolation and metabolic characteristics of rat and chicken enterocytes. *Biochem J* 1979 ; 178 : 589-96.
17. Clausen MR, Mortensen PB. Kinetic studies on the metabolism of short-chain fatty acids and glucose by isolated rat colonocytes. *Gastroenterology* 1994 ; 106 : 423-32.
18. Fleming SE, Fitch MD, De Vries S, Liu ML, Kight C. Nutrient utilization by cells isolated from rat jejunum, cecum and colon. *J Nutr* 1991 ; 121 : 869-78.
19. Ardawi MS, Newsholme EA. Fuel utilization in colonocytes of the rat. *Biochem J* 1985 ; 231 : 713-9.
20. Darcy-Vrillon B, Morel MT, Cherbuy C, Bernard F, Posho L, Blachier F, Meslin JC, Duée PH. Metabolic characteristics of pig colonocytes after adaptation to a high fiber diet. *J Nutr* 1993 ; 123 : 234-43.
21. Roediger WEW, Duncan A, Kapaniris O, Millard S. Reducing sulfur compounds of the colon impair colonocyte nutrition : implications for ulcerative colitis. *Gastroenterology* 1993 ; 104 : 802-9.
22. Cherbuy C, Darcy-Vrillon B, Morel MT, Borlet A, Blachier F, Duée PH. Metabolic characteristics of isolated colonocytes : modulation by dietary fibre or by the colonic microflora. *Proc Nutr Soc* 1993 ; 52 : 133 A.
23. Demigné C, Yacoub C, Rémésy C. Effects of absorption of large amounts of volatile fatty acids on rat liver metabolism. *J Nutr* 1986 ; 116 : 77-86.
24. Morand C, Rémésy C, Levrat MA, Demigné C. Replacement of digestible wheat starch by resistant corn starch alters splanchnic metabolism in rats. *J Nutr* 1992 ; 122 : 345-54.
25. Morand C, Levrat MA, Besson C, Demigné C, Rémésy C. Effects of a diet rich in resistant starch on hepatic lipid metabolism in the rat. *J Nutr Biochem* 1994 ; 5 : 138-44.
26. Demigné C, Rémésy C. Hepatic metabolism of short-chain fatty acids. In : Roche AF, ed. *Short chain fatty acids : metabolism and clinical importance.* Report of the 10th Ross Conference on Medical Research. Colombus, Ohio : Ross Laboratories, 1991 : 17-23.
27. Scholte HR, Groot PHE. Organ and intra-cellular localization of short chain acyl-CoA synthetases in rat and guinea-pig. *Biochim Biophys Acta* 1975 ; 409 : 283-96.
28. Crabtree B, Gordon MJ, Christie SL. Measurement of the rates of acetyl-CoA hydrolysis and synthesis from acetate in rat hepatocytes and the role of these fluxes in substrate cycling. *Biochem J* 1990 ; 270 : 219-25.
29. Anderson JW, Bridges SR. Short-chain fatty acid fermentation products of plant fiber affect glucose metabolism of isolated rat hepatocytes. *Proc Soc Exp Biol Med* 1984 ; 177 : 372-6.
30. Duée PH, Pégorier JP, El Manoubi L, Ferré P, Bois-Joyeux B, Girard J. Development of gluconeogenesis from different substrates in newborn rabbit hepatocytes. *J Dev Physiol* 1986 ; 8 : 387-94.

31. Demigné C, Yacoub C, Rémésy C, Fafournoux P. Propionate and butyrate metabolism in rat or sheep hepatocytes. *Biochim Biophys Acta* 1986 ; 875 : 535-42.
32. Chan TM, Freedland RA. The effect of propionate on the metabolism of pyruvate and lactate in the perfused rat liver. *Biochem J 1972 ; 127 : 539-43.*
33. *Chen WJL, Anderson JW, Jennings D. Propionate may mediate the hypocholesterolemic effects of certain soluble plant fibers in cholesterol fed rats. Proc Soc Exp Biol Med 1984 ; 175 : 215-8.*
34. Nishina PM, Freedland RA. Effects of propionate on lipid biosynthesis in isolated rat hepatocytes. *J Nutr* 1990 ; 120 : 668-73.
35. Wright RS, Anderson JW, Bridges SR. Propionate inhibits hepatocyte lipid synthesis. *Proc Soc Exp Biol Med* 1990 ; 195 : 26-9.
36. Scheppach W, Cummings JH, Branch WJ, Schrezenmeir J. Effect of gut-derived acetate on oral glucose tolerance in man. *Clin Sci* 1988 ; 75 : 355-61.
37. Scheppach W, Wiggins HS, Halliday D, Self R, Howard J, Branch WJ, Schrezenmeir J, Cummings JH. Effet of gut-derived acetate on glucose turnover in man. *Clin Sci* 1988 ; 363-70.
38. Laurent C, Paichard C, Marks L, Baschi S, Champ M, Charbonnel B, Krempf M. Effect of short chain fatty acids on hepatic glucose production in humans. *Am J Clin Nutr* 1995 (in press).
39. Topping DL. Soluble fiber polysaccharides : effects on plasma cholesterol and colonic fermentation. *Nutr Rev* 1991 ; 49 : 195-203.

Achevé d'imprimer par Corlet, Imprimeur, S.A.
14110 Condé-sur-Noireau (France)
N° d'Imprimeur : 9921 - Dépôt légal : juin 1995

Imprimé en C.E.E.